FRAMING THE
SEXUAL SUBJECT

FRAMING THE SEXUAL SUBJECT

The Politics of
Gender, Sexuality, and Power

Edited by

RICHARD PARKER,

REGINA MARIA BARBOSA,

AND PETER AGGLETON

UNIVERSITY OF CALIFORNIA PRESS
BERKELEY   LOS ANGELES   LONDON

University of California Press
Berkeley and Los Angeles, California

University of California Press, Ltd.
London, England

© 2000 by
The Regents of the University of California

Framing the sexual subject : the politics of gender, sexuality, and
    power / edited by Richard Parker, Regina Maria Barbosa, and Peter
    Aggleton.
        p.   cm.
    Includes bibliographical references and index.
    ISBN 0-520-21836-1 (cloth : alk. paper). — ISBN 0-520-21838-8
(pbk. : alk. paper)
    1. Sex—Political aspects, cross-cultural studies.   2. Sex role—
Political aspects, cross-cultural studies.   3. Power (Social
sciences), cross-cultural studies.   4. AIDS (Disease)—Patients—
Civil rights, cross-cultural studies.   I. Parker, Richard G.
(Richard Guy), 1956–   .   II. Barbosa, Regina Maria.   III. Aggleton,
Peter.
HQ23.F76   2000
305.3—dc21   99-38466
                                                              CIP

Printed in the United States of America
9 8 7 6 5 4 3 2 1

The paper used in this publication meets the minimum
requirements of American National Standard for Information
Sciences—Permanence of Paper for Printed Library Materials,
ANSI Z39.48-1984.

In memory of
Jonathan M. Mann
1947–1998

Contents

Part Three: Hegemony, Oppression, and Empowerment

Acknowledgments

This book would not have been possible without the contribution of many institutions and individuals. It brings together a number of the papers originally presented at a conference in Rio de Janeiro in 1996, organized by the Program on Gender, Sexuality, and Health at the Center for Research and Study in Collective Health (CEPESC) of the Institute of Social Medicine (IMS), State University of Rio de Janeiro (UERJ), with support provided by the Ford Foundation and the John D. and Catherine T. MacArthur Foundation.

For their help in preparing the manuscript, we would particularly like to thank Ana Paula Uziel, Juan Carlos de la Concepción Raxach, Vagner de Almeida, and Rita Rizzo at the Institute of Social Medicine; Charles Klein, Delia Easton, and Chris White at the HIV Center for Clinical and Behavioral Studies, New York State Psychiatric Institute and Columbia University; and Helen Thomas and Paula Hassett at the Thomas Coram Research Unit, Institute of Education, University of London.

The final manuscript has also benefitted greatly from suggestions by the three outside reviewers who commented for the University of California Press: Margaret Connors, Jonathan Mann, and Steve Epstein. Those suggestions were crucial in revising and rethinking the volume.

We particularly wish to dedicate the book to Jonathan Mann, whose tragic death occurred as we were finalizing our work. Jonathan was both friend and mentor to many of the editors and contributors. As most readers will know, he was tireless in his work against the HIV/ AIDS pandemic and for health and human rights. What many may not know is that he was also fundamentally committed to research on sexuality and sexual health. His work as founding director of the World Health Organization's Global Programme on AIDS had convinced him that one of the greatest barriers to responding to the HIV/ AIDS epidemic globally was the remarkable silence, stigma, and discrimination so often associated with issues related to gender and sexuality around the world. When he left WHO and moved to Harvard University to found the François-Xavier Bagnoud Center for Health and Human Rights, he worked with Richard Parker to create an international working group on sexuality research that is in many ways the direct precursor to the project leading to the current volume and involved many of its contributors—and he continued to support and defend sex research until his untimely death. His was, as Rosalind Petchesky, one of the contributors to this volume, put it, "a vital and powerful voice for what we are all working for." He will be sorely missed.

Introduction

Framing the Sexual Subject

Richard Parker, Regina Maria Barbosa,
and Peter Aggleton

For the greater part of the twentieth century, human sexuality was largely ignored as a focus for social research and reflection. Perhaps because the experience of sexuality seems so intimately linked to our bodies, it was relatively easy to relegate the subject matter of sexuality to the realm of the biomedical sciences, where it became the focus for obscure medical tomes and arcane psychiatric practices but seemed to have little to do with the more crucial and immediate problems of social life. Indeed, only in recent years, during the closing decades of the century, has this marginalization of sexuality and its submission to the biomedical gaze begun to give way to a more far-reaching social and political analysis. And it is only over the course of the last decade, from the mid-1980s to the mid-1990s, that a veritable boom in social research on sexuality seems to have taken place (Parker and Gagnon, 1995).[1]

The reasons for this recent explosion of interest are of course complex and diverse. They clearly have much to do with a set of reconfigurations taking place in the social sciences more broadly in the late twentieth century, as disciplines such as history, sociology, and anthropology have struggled to find new ways of understanding the rapidly changing postmodern world, placing new emphasis on domains once considered relatively "private"—that is, outside the realm of serious social scientific investigation—but increasingly understood as socially shaped (Vance, 1991). Perhaps most important, this growing attention to sexuality as a key field for social analysis has been mandated by a set of changes within society itself since the 1960s, including the growing feminist and gay and lesbian movements and their impact on academic disciplines, university practices, and even, in

1

some instances, government policies (Parker and Gagnon, 1995; see also Lancaster and di Leonardo, 1997).

At the same time that these social movements have been crucial in calling attention to questions of gender and sexuality, growing international concern with issues such as over population, reproductive health, and, perhaps especially, the emerging HIV/AIDS pandemic, has intersected with the research agendas constructed around feminist and gay and lesbian concerns. Indeed, while social and moral conservatives might have preferred to dismiss questions related to gender, sexuality, and sexual rights as little more than the private concerns of progressive (or "perverse") minorities, the broader social implications of global issues of overpopulation, reproductive health, and AIDS have guaranteed that the study of sexuality, and of its social and political dimensions, would necessarily emerge as central to many important debates taking place in late-twentieth-century society (Corrêa, 1994; Ginsberg and Rapp, 1995; Lancaster and di Leonardo, 1997; Parker and Gagnon, 1995; Petchesky and Judd, 1998).

As part of broader global social change, these emerging issues have taken shape at a moment when many boundaries between the so-called developed and developing worlds (and their social, political, and intellectual concerns) have broken down—or at the very least blurred—bringing what may once have been different currents into increasing contact and creating dialogue around issues of sexuality and politics on a truly transnational scale. Feminist concepts and gay, lesbian, and queer theory have become moving forces behind research and social movements in many developing countries; the impact of structural violence in shaping HIV/AIDS vulnerability and a range of reproductive health problems has become as apparent in the cities of the First World as in those of the Third; reproductive and sexual rights movements have taken on global dimensions; and demarcations between academic researchers and social and political activists have become increasingly unclear. Ultimately, the current volume situates itself, as do most of the researchers represented here, within a broader rethinking of issues related to gender, sexuality, and power in the late twentieth century. The book seeks to contribute to the growing dialogue taking place today both north and south of the equator (Parker, 1999) about the social organization of sexual experience and the social imagination of the sexual subject—a sexual subject that is both the *subject-matter* for politically committed investigation and the *subject-agent* of conscious struggles for social and sexual change.

Shifting Paradigms

It is important to remember that this interconnected set of concerns has not always been dominant, or indeed even present, in much research carried out on sexuality, particularly in relation to health, even in quite recent times. On the contrary, the concerns most strongly represented here might be described as something of an alternative current, evolving in important ways over time but nonetheless largely marginal (and often marginalized) in relation to the approaches that have tended to dominate the general field of sexuality research (in terms of both research funding and institutional legitimacy). Indeed, throughout much of the twentieth century, sexological research (and similar approaches presenting themselves as objective "sciences" of sexual life) have largely avoided direct engagement with politics, as if avoiding the subject might somehow spare sex researchers from engaging in political debate, leaving them safe in their laboratories to continue seeking "natural truths" of sexual function.[2] Even with the veritable explosion in sexuality research since the mid-1980s—particularly as a consequence of the global HIV/AIDS pandemic—the vast majority of research attention has focused less on the kinds of political questions considered in the current volume than on a far narrower attempt to construct a science of sexual behavior valid independent of vagaries of time and place, much less of the shifting sands of political struggle.

The problematic epistemological and political status of such a scientific project had of course been obvious for some time—unmasked and critiqued by feminist, and by gay and lesbian, studies seeking to deconstruct the working of scientific discourse in relation to gender and sexuality so as to uncover the relations between knowledge and power within the sexual field (see for example Foucault, 1978; Snitow, Stansell, and Thompson, 1983; Weeks, 1985; Vance, 1984, 1991). While the gradual but progressive demedicalization of sexuality in social research had been an important achievement of "social constructionist" approaches since the late 1970s and early 1980s, there can be little doubt about the profound remedicalization of sexuality in the wake of the HIV/AIDS pandemic (Vance, 1991; Parker and

Easton, 1998). Indeed, much social research activity that emerged in response to AIDS in the mid-1980s focused not on the social construction of sexual experience, let alone its political dimensions, but on surveys of risk-related behavior and on the knowledge, attitudes, and practices that might be associated with the risk of HIV infection. Most studies sought to collect quantifiable data on sexual partners, specific sexual practices, sexually transmitted diseases (STDs), and similar factors understood to contribute to the spread of HIV—and, on the basis of this documentation, to point the way for policies and intervention programs aimed at reducing behavioral risk of infection (see for example Carballo, Cleland, Caraël, and Albrecht, 1989; Chouinard and Albert, 1989; Turner, Miller, and Moses, 1989; Cleland and Ferry, 1995).

Particularly in the United States, a longstanding focus on "behavioral" research in public health on what were understood as individualistic determinants of "health behaviors" and on what was believed a rational decision-making process associated with "behavioral change" in response to perceived health threats, meant that many of the earliest research initiatives in response to the HIV/AIDS epidemic were designed to provide an empirical basis for "behavioral interventions" (understood as a social equivalent to surgical or biomedical interventions in the physiological body) aimed at modifying activities understood as posing the risk of infection.[3] Based on theoretical models such as the Health Belief Model (Becker and Joseph, 1988), Theory of Reasoned Action (Ajzen and Fishbein, 1980), and Social Learning Theory (Bandura, 1977), "intervention research" aimed to produce behavioral change by providing members of target population groups with adequate knowledge and information about the risk of HIV infection, and by increasing their perception and awareness of such risk, to stimulate the rational decision-making process believed to lead ultimately to significant risk reduction. It was assumed that, by focusing on links between sexual behavior and individual psychology, more broad-based prevention programs could eventually be developed, based upon further intervention research findings, to persuade individuals to change their behaviors so as to not only reduce HIV infection risk but also make it possible to respond to other problems presumed linked to sexual conduct, such as the spread of other STDs, the epidemics of teenage pregnancy in the inner cities of industrialized countries, and the population explosion believed taking place in the developing world (see for example Turner, Miller, and Moses, 1990; Turner, Miller, and Moses, 1989; Bancroft, 1997).

While this basic approach was most pronounced in the United States (where the size of the HIV/AIDS epidemic, the availability of resources, and the individualistic behavioral research tradition were also most pronounced), similar initiatives took place throughout the 1980s and early 1990s in many parts of the Anglo-European world and—particularly under the auspices of bilateral or intergovernmental agencies such as USAID and the World Health Organization—in a growing number of developing countries in Africa, Asia, and Latin America (Carballo, Cleland, Caraël, and Albrecht, 1989; Cleland and Ferry, 1995; see also the discussion in Aggleton, 1996b). Increasingly, however, as behavioral research and behavioral interventions developed in a growing range of social and cultural settings, the relative effectiveness of research instruments and intervention strategies came into question. The difficulties of translating or adapting research protocols for cross-cultural application quickly became apparent, in the face of often radically different understandings of sexual expression and drug use in different societies and even in different subcultures of a broader society (Aggleton, 1996b; Parker, 1994). And the inefficacy of behavioral interventions based on information and reasoned persuasion to stimulate risk reduction became evident almost immediately. Study after study showed that information, in and of itself, was insufficient to produce risk-reducing behavioral change, and the relative limitations of using individual psychology as the basis for intervention and prevention programs became (even in the United States) apparent (Aggleton, 1996b; Cohen, 1991; Parker, 1994, 1996). By the late 1980s, therefore, on the basis both of research findings and of practical experience around the world, it was becoming clear that a far more complex set of social, structural, and cultural factors mediate the structure of risk in every population group, and that the dynamics of individual psychology could never explain (or stimulate) changes in sexual conduct without taking these broader issues into account (Aggleton, 1996b; Aggleton and Coates, 1995; Parker, 1994, 1996; Sweat and Dennison, 1995; Watney, 1990).

By the late 1980s and early 1990s, a range of broader forces had begun to be understood as central to a more adequate understanding of the social dimensions of the HIV and AIDS epidemic, as well as of related aspects of sexual health; at the same time, the limitations of traditional behavioral research approaches were becoming apparent, particularly with regard to developing interventions. Strongly influenced by changes within interactionist sociology and cultural anthropology, by moves to radicalize social psychology, and by insights from new fields such as women's studies and gay and lesbian studies, attention turned to the broader social and cultural structures and meanings shaping or constructing sexual experience in given settings. Stimulated by social constructionist concerns, an important shift began from a focus on individual psychology to a new concern with intersubjective cultural meanings related to sexuality, and with their shared and collective qualities not as the property of atomized or isolated individuals, but of social persons integrated within distinct, and diverse, cultures. Such research has increasingly sought to go beyond calculation of behavioral frequencies and identification of statistical correlates of sexual risk behavior to examine what sex *means* to the parties involved, the contexts in which it takes place, the structure and scripting of sexual encounters, and the sexual cultures (and subcultures) present and emergent within particular societies (see for example Aggleton, 1996b; Herdt and Lindenbaum, 1992; Kippax and Crawford, 1993; Parker, 1994, 1995; Parker, Herdt, and Carballo, 1991).[4]

The focus of much important sexuality research over the past decade has thus moved from behavior to the cultural settings within which behavior takes place—and to the cultural rules that organize behavior (Parker and Aggleton, 1999). Special emphasis has been given to analyzing the indigenous cultural categories and classification systems that structure and define sexual experience in different social and cultural contexts. It has become increasingly apparent that many key categories and classifications (such as "homosexuality" or "prostitution") hitherto used to describe sexual behaviors in Western medicine and public health epidemiology are far from universal—and far from unchanging in meaning even where they exist (see for example Alonso and Koreck, 1989; Aggleton, 1996a; Daniel and Parker, 1993; Herdt, 1997; Herdt and Lindenbaum, 1992; Lancaster, 1992, 1995, 1997; Parker and Aggleton, 1999; Parker, 1994, 1995; Parker and Carballo, 1990; Parker, Herdt, and Carballo, 1990; Patton, 1990; de Zalduondo, 1991). By focusing more carefully on local categories and classifications, the cultural analysis of sexual meanings has sought to move from what, in anthropology or linguistics, might be described as an "outsider" perspective to what is described as an "insider" perspective—and from the "experience-distant" concepts of science to the "experience-near" concepts that members of specific cultures use to understand and interpret their own reality (Geertz, 1983; Parker, 1989, 1991, 1994, 1995).

This shift of emphasis from study of individual behaviors to research on cultural meanings has drawn attention to the socially constructed identities and communities structuring sexual practice within collective life (Aggleton, 1996b; Kippax and Crawford, 1993; Parker, 1991, 1994, 1995). On the basis of such work, an important reformulation of the very notion of intervention has begun—indeed, it has become increasingly apparent that the idea of "behavioral intervention" may be a misnomer, that preventive interventions almost never function at the level of behavior but, rather, at the level of social or collective representations, and that new knowledge about perceived sexual risk is always necessarily interpreted within the context of pre-existing systems of meaning, which mediate the incorporation of such information into action (Kippax and Crawford, 1993; Parker, 1994, 1995). Precisely because action has increasingly come to be understood as socially constructed and collective, earlier forms of behavioral intervention have increasingly given way to community based, culturally grounded, education and prevention programs aimed at transforming norms and values and reconstituting collective meanings to effectively promote safer sexual practices (Aggleton, 1996b; Kippax, Connell, Dowsett, and Crawford, 1993; Parker, 1994, 1996).

While the work emerging on the social and cultural construction of sexual meanings has thus provided important new insights on the factors shaping sexual health, and has increasingly offered the basis for more culturally sensitive, community based programs, it has also become evident that the factors influencing the construction of sexual realities are more complex than originally perceived, and that the social, cultural, political, and economic dimensions of sexual life are more complicated than once imagined. Perhaps in consequence, attention has more fully focused on the ways different communities structure the possibilities of sexual interaction, thereby defining a given range of potential sexual partners and practices. Whom one is permitted to have sex with, in what ways, under what circumstances, and with what specific outcomes are never random; such possibilities are defined through explicit and implicit rules imposed by the sexual

cultures of specific communities, and by the underlying power relations. This increasing awareness of the ways sexual communities structure the possibilities of sexual contact has drawn special attention to
socially and culturally sanctioned differentials in power—particularly
between men and women (see for example de Zalduondo and Bernard, 1995; Rao Gupta and Weiss, 1995; Heise, 1995; Lancaster, 1992;
Parker, 1991; Parker and Barbosa, 1996; Stein, 1990), but also, in
some instances, between different types of men (see Aggleton, 1996a;
Lancaster, 1992, 1995, 1997; Parker, 1991, 1999; Prieur, 1998).

Because sexual cultures organize sexual inequality in specific ways,
cultural rules and regulations place specific limitations on the potential for negotiation in sexual interactions—and in turn condition the
possibilities for sexual violence, for patterns of contraceptive use, for
HIV/AIDS risk-reduction strategies, and so on. The dynamics of gender power relations have thus become a major focus for contemporary
research, particularly in relation to reproductive health and to the
rapid spread of HIV infection among women in many parts of the
world (see for example Ginsberg and Rapp, 1995; Rao Gupta and
Weiss, 1995; Heise, 1995; Parker and Gagnon, 1995).

This increasing confrontation with issues of power, and with the
relationship between culture and power, has forced social research
on sexuality to address broader structural issues than previously—
issues that, in interaction with culturally constituted systems of meaning, play a key role in organizing the sexual field and defining the
possibilities open to sexual subjects (Parker and Easton, 1998). New
theoretical approaches are reaching beyond postmodernism, while
still embracing postmodernist problematizations of sex, gender, race,
and class, to offer more grounded and politically relevant research
agenda within the context of rapid social change characterizing the
processes of late-twentieth-century globalization (see, in particular,
Harvey, 1990. See specifically in relation to sex research, Lancaster,
1995, 1997; Parker and Gagnon, 1995; Parker, 1999).

Work casting the body as both a symbolic and a material product
of culture has provided an especially important way of reframing recent sexuality research (see for example Lancaster, 1992; Parker,
1999; Bishop and Robinson, 1998). Engaged activist research in response to AIDS, for instance, has insisted upon the necessity of
evaluating class and ethnicity (see for example Dowsett, 1996; Patton,
1990; Watney, 1994; and Treichler, 1992). More broadly, a growing

critical literature has begun to emerge examining colonialism and neo-colonialism as contexts of power shaping regimes of sexuality (see for example Hyam, 1990; Manderson and Jolly, 1997; Stoler, 1995; Young, 1995). Contextualizing sexuality within political economy has underscored how extensively prevailing notions about sexuality, gender, and desire are fueled by a colonialist mentality that presumes a cross-cultural rigidity and consistency of sexual categories and the durability of geographic and cultural boundaries imposed by Western scholars (Manderson and Jolly, 1997; Parker and Gagnon, 1995; Parker and Easton, 1998). One key challenge confronting sexuality research has thus emerged as the urgent need to rethink the effects of colonialism and neo-colonialism not only on the construction of sexuality (both North and South), but on the ways research has been conducted and the voices that have been allowed to speak. Perhaps most important, a new wave of researchers working from a range of subaltern contexts has begun to make itself heard: feminist, and gay and lesbian, researchers, to be sure, but increasingly researchers not only from the Northern, Anglo-European world, but also from the countries and cultures of Africa, Asia, and Latin America.

By the mid-1990s, then, just as social and cultural analysis emerged as an important corrective to the perceived limitations of earlier behavioral approaches, a new focus on political and economic analysis of the factors associated with the social construction of sexual experience, and structuring the possibilities for social and sexual change, thus emerged as central to an evolving field of research focusing on gender, sexuality, and power in the contemporary world. Taken together, such recent studies have also suggested important reformulations in the ways research might feed into intervention, prevention activities, and struggles for political and social change. Perhaps most important, the studies have called attention to the community base necessary for intervention programs, and to the importance of understanding the relationship between sexuality and health in political as well as technical terms. They have also brought attention to the need for structural and environmental programs and activities aimed at transforming the broader social, cultural, political, and economic forces that structure vulnerability (whether to unwanted pregnancy, HIV infection, or sexual oppression and violence), and at enabling members of affected communities to respond more adequately to these forces (Aggleton, 1996b; Sweat and Dennison, 1995; Parker,

1996). In particular, such studies have focused attention on the extent to which struggles for sexual health and sexual well-being, like struggles for sexual rights and sexual citizenship, in cultures around the world must be understood as part of broader processes of social transformation aimed not merely at the reduction of sexual risks but at the redress of social and economic inequality and injustice (Altman 1994; Parker, 1996; Parker and Barbosa, 1996).

The Politics of Gender, Sexuality, and Power

Taken together, these recent developments in sexuality research, and growing interest on a range of issues impacting the politics of sexuality in specific communities, as well as at a global level, provide the background and foundation for the essays brought together here. While the various chapters explore a range of directions and theoretical perspectives, they are united by a common concern to understand the rapidly changing shape of sex and sexuality around the globe as the twentieth century draws to a close, and by commitment to apply this understanding to concrete struggles for sexual rights, health, and well-being. Through their contributions, the authors seek to reconfigure existing notions of gender and sexuality so as to link them more effectively to understandings of power, resistance, and emancipation. The concept of the sexual subject (and of sexual subjectivity) as a focus not only for investigation but also for action (HIV/AIDS prevention, sexual and reproductive rights advocacy, or related programs of social change) thus lies at the very heart of these texts—and is central to the more general and collective intellectual and political project to which this volume seeks to contribute.

In organizing *Framing the Sexual Subject*, we have divided the chapters into three major parts that reflect not only the major research directions present in the essays themselves but also three of the most productive areas of current work in the field. Part One, "Bodies, Cultures, and Identities," derives from a research tradition informed by social constructionist approaches in gay and lesbian studies, but seeks to reframe and recontextualize questions of sexual identity in new and important ways. In chapter 1, "Bodyplay: Corporeality in a Discursive Silence," for example, Gary W. Dowsett builds upon recent work in postmodern theory and criticism to rethink not merely the social construction of sexual identities but the sexual construction of society itself. By focusing on the erotic body and its sexual practices, and by exploring what he describes as the "relationality" of gay sex, Dowsett draws powerfully on his own positioned experience as both researcher and gay man, and seeks to move beyond the reductionisms of a simplistic positivist sexology, as well as of an overly mechanistic social constructionism in which sexuality emerges as little more than the product of social relations. He argues for a more complex, nuanced understanding of sociality as produced through the enactment of desire—and, by placing sexuality at the center of the creation of sociality, opens new possibilities for understanding the sexual construction of social space, of identities and subjectivities, of desiring collectivities and sexual cultures.

In chapter 2, "Masculinity in Indonesia: Genders, Sexualities, and Identities in a Changing Society," Dédé Oetomo focuses on male sexualities and sexual cultures in Indonesia, examining the complex ways the construction of masculinity takes place, not only vis-à-vis women and femininity, but also in relation to the *waria* gender category and to a variety of types of men who, whether homosexually identified or not, have sex with men. Developing, like Dowsett, an engaged reading of gender based heavily on his own experience as both an academic and a gay activist, Oetomo is able to expand upon the significant attention given to "third gender" categories in much recent anthropological and cross-cultural research (see for example Garber, 1992; Herdt, 1993; Nanda, 1985, and the critiques in Kulick, 1998, and Prieur, 1998). He can move beyond the obvious risks of objectifying and exoticizing alternative gender realities—the risk, for instance, of adding them as yet another in our collection of exotic sexual butterflies—precisely because he can speak from his own situated position within Indonesian society, and is able to use the *waria* category to illuminate broader interactive patterns in the construction of gendered subjectivities in Indonesian culture. Oetomo demonstrates the extent to which gender power and sexual domination are not simply a function of gender differences in what he describes as "the mainstream sense," but are functions of class distinctions, age differences, and unequal power relations in society.

In the last essay of this section, chapter 3, "Male Homosexuality and Seropositivity: The Construction of Social Identities in Brazil," Veriano Terto Jr. extends recent work on emerging homosexual and gay identities and communities in countries such as Brazil (see for example Parker, 1999; Parker and Terto Jr., 1998), to examine how these new forms have been linked to the experience of HIV infection and the construction of seropositivity as a discrete social/sexual identity. Nowhere over the past two decades has the history of homosexuality evolved entirely separate from the HIV/AIDS epidemic; while complex and diverse gay communities existed previously in the Anglo-European world, in many parts of the developing world the emergence of gay identities and communities has been largely contemporaneous with the emergence and evolution of AIDS. This fact has shaped social response to the epidemic and the cultural politics of homosexuality in highly specific ways. By drawing heavily, like Dowsett and Oetomo, on long experience not only as a researcher but also as both a gay and an AIDS activist, and by examining the social organization of homosexuality in Brazil prior to and following the emergence of AIDS, Terto is able to highlight the myriad ways the epidemic has transformed the subjective experience of homosexual men. He shows how research on the impact of AIDS on homosexually active men has led to a fuller understanding of the latter's impact on the course of the epidemic—of how gay men and emerging gay communities have affected Brazilian society's responses to AIDS, and how this contribution has itself influenced reconstruction of social representations of the epidemic and themselves.

While the chapters in Part One build heavily on a broader body of work in gay and lesbian studies and HIV/AIDS research, the three texts in Part Two, "Sex, Gender, and Power," link both fields to work in feminist theory and gender studies, and to a growing concern with the global dimensions of gender inequality and its consequences for sexual health and sexual rights. Although an extensive body of theoretical and empirical work has been produced on questions of gender and power in recent decades (for just a few key examples, see Butler, 1990; Haraway, 1991; Rubin, 1975, 1984; Scott, 1986; Vance, 1984), much of this work has focused on the Anglo-European world; the incorporation of such perspectives in cross-cultural research and analysis has proven rather more difficult. While important attempts at comparative analysis have been made, and cross-cultural documentation of gender inequalities has been extensive (see for example Heise, 1995; Rao Gupta and Weiss, 1995), comparative research has often been limited to repeated generalizations and found it hard to move on to more nuanced cross-cultural understanding of the structures that organize gender inequality, the processes through which it is concretely negotiated, and the ways possibly to intervene effectively against it. The papers in Part Two seek to address these key dilemmas, although in distinct, but complementary, ways: through an analysis of possibilities of, and barriers to global political processes and coalitions; through comparative, cross-national investigation; and through detailed analysis of local contexts as a point of departure for design of more effective intervention and service provision.

Questions related to global political processes and struggles for reproductive and sexual rights are central to Rosalind Petchesky's analysis in chapter 4, "Sexual Rights: Inventing a Concept, Mapping an International Practice." Building on work carried out with her colleagues in the International Reproductive Rights Research Action Group (a collaborative international team of feminist researchers and activists from Brazil, Egypt, Malaysia, Mexico, Nigeria, the Philippines, and the United States), Petchesky argues that sexual rights can be described as "the newest kid on the block in international debates about the meaning and practices of human rights." Prior to 1993, no international instrument relevant to human rights made reference to sexuality or sexual rights—the idea of sexual rights simply did not exist as part of international human rights discourse. An important turning point came in 1993 with the World Conference on Human Rights in Vienna, where the Declaration and Programme of Action, responding to intensive efforts of the women's human rights lobby, called for the elimination of gender-based violence, sexual harassment, and exploitation. It was only in 1994, however, at the International Conference on Population and Development in Cairo, that sex, sexuality, and sexual health began to enter international debates not merely in relation to violence and violation but as a positive part of human experience to be preserved and nurtured. For the first time in any international policy document, the ICPD Programme of Action explicitly included "sexual health" in an array of rights that population and development programs should protect. Yet even here, extension of such rights was ambiguous at best, linked first and foremost to heterosexual reproduction. Again, in 1995, the Platform for Action of the Fourth World Women's Conference in Beijing, after much struggle and debate, reconfirmed the commitment to reproductive rights that had emerged in Cairo, but without reference (in the final document) to either sexual rights or sexual orientation. Ultimately, then, Petchesky argues, in spite of the intensive efforts of the international women's movement, and of the much smaller yet important international lesbian and gay rights movement, even by the mid-1990s it was still largely impossible to develop an affirmative approach to sexual rights within the broader context of the international human rights movement. At best, there has been a focus on the oppression and violence suffered by women (and to a lesser extent sexual minorities) around the world—part of a "reactive" response to the plight of sexual victims. We have failed, moreover, to develop a more affirmative and emancipatory notion of sexual rights (transcending medical and technical problematics) as a social good fundamental to any adequate notion of human well-being and dignity.

Many of these dilemmas over how gender relations are to be conceived and transformed without linking notions of sexual health to a conception of sexual rights as fundamental to human dignity are equally evident in studies of gender power in the context of the HIV/AIDS pandemic. In chapter 5, "Cross-National Perspectives on Gender and Power," Purnima Mane and Peter Aggleton report on research that they initiated under the auspices of the World Health Organization's Global Programme on AIDS (with later support by the Joint United Nations Programme on HIV/AIDS). Working in collaboration with investigators from Costa Rica, Indonesia, Mexico, and Senegal, they aimed to examine prevailing gender relations, patterns and processes of sexual communication, and the capacity of the female condom to empower women in sexual "negotiations" with men. Mane and Aggleton argue convincingly for a participatory approach to implementing interventions aimed at introducing new prevention methods, suggesting that empowerment through use of such methods may best be thought of as a process along a continuum, rather than as an all-or-nothing alternative. They stress the structural factors impinging on the lives of women engaged in sex work compared with those not in such work and argue for recognition that it is not simply the availability of new technologies that must be guaranteed, but the collective support for their adoption within the context of ongoing dialogue on the structure of gender relations and the impact of this structure on women's lives.

In chapter 6, "Gender Stereotypes and Power Relations: Unacknowledged Risks for STDs in Argentina," Mónica Gogna and Silvina

Ramos shift the focus from cross-national comparisons to a detailed discussion of gender and power in the specific setting of urban Buenos Aires, and the implications of existing culturally constituted gender relations for effective reproductive health service provision. Building on a long tradition of feminist and reproductive health research, and focusing on the importance of understanding how individuals and groups perceive, conceptualize, and find meaning in their social and physical worlds, Gogna and Ramos analyze the cultural and psychosocial forces that construct STDs at the point of intersection of three significantly different cultural domains—health/illness, sexuality, and gender—demonstrating the ways conceptions and prescriptions from these domains reinforce and neutralize one another. They argue that STDs are rooted in concepts of gender identities and sexual meanings (related to pleasure, sin, and reproduction, among others) in ways that profoundly affect both prevention and treatment, limiting the possibilities for interventions that fail to take such factors into account, and they examine the implications of these concepts for the provision of health care services seeking to more effectively meet the needs of both women and men.

Taken together, the chapters in Part Two provide a unique view of the linkages and interactions between global processes and local social and cultural contexts in the late twentieth century. They offer a clear sense of the ways international agencies and the intergovernmental system, national governments and programs, and local level services and cultures must be examined to build greater understanding of the challenges and struggles that today organize gender and sexuality in relation to sexual health and sexual rights. Many of these concerns are also present, though in somewhat different ways, in Part Three, "Hegemony, Oppression, and Empowerment," in four chapters examining the ways multiple forms of sexual oppression are articulated and constructed through different cultural, social, and economic systems, as well as the possibilities and barriers for the empowerment of sexual subjects within such settings.

In chapter 7, "AIDS, Medicine, and Moral Panic in the Philippines," Michael Tan examines the ways AIDS discourse has taken shape in the media and popular culture in the Philippines to produce a sense of sexual difference synonymous with moral and physical danger. Tracing the construction of HIV and AIDS through the Philippine press, Tan analyzes what he describes as "the medico-moral hegemony" that is produced and reproduced at the level of collective representations, and that shapes the response to AIDS not only by far-right conservative groups but also by government and even many non-governmental AIDS-service organizations. He suggests that most HIV prevention campaigns in the Philippines have been based on longstanding and highly problematic models of "social hygiene" that today, as in the past, structure the reaction of the public health system to notions of sexual diversity and difference—and that legitimize public health practices of surveillance and control.

In chapter 8, "Survival Sex and HIV/AIDS in an African City," the emphasis on cultural hegemony and control shifts slightly to examination of the political economy of sexual oppression, as Eleanor Preston-Whyte, Christine Varga, Herman Oosthuizen, Rachel Roberts, and Frederick Blose map the diverse social and cultural spaces of female and male sex work, and explore the intersecting structures of economic marginalization, racism, sexism, and heterosexism that shape the possibilities for risk reduction on the part of sex workers in Durban, South Africa. While sex work and sex workers have become the objects of biomedical and epidemiological research in the wake of the HIV/AIDS pandemic, this research has often treated them as little more than vectors of infection and danger (see, in particular, the critique in de Zalduondo, 1991; see also Aggleton, 1998). Indeed, the study of sex work has too often ignored the objective conditions that organize it, and the diverse forms of "structural violence" (Farmer, Connors, and Simmons, 1996) that typically confront sex workers. This neglect has in turn made it almost impossible to intervene in meaningful ways to reduce both behavioral risk and social vulnerability. Against this backdrop, Preston-Whyte and her colleagues focus on the ways diverse forms of sex work in different parts of Durban take shape as part of a broader range of survival strategies by poor and marginalized women and men—who must daily confront a spectrum of intersecting oppressions to make ends meet in a context of unprecedented social and political change. The authors' analysis points to urgent need for both a more general political economy of sex work and the implementation of structural and environmental interventions capable of confronting the factors organizing behavioral risk and systematically denying men and women engaged in sex work their most fundamental rights and dignity.

Confronting the denial is also a central concern in chapter 9, "Cultural Regulation, Self-Regulation, and Sexuality: A Psycho-Cultural Model of HIV Risk in Latino Gay Men," by Rafael Diaz, which focuses on interrelated social and cultural factors that impact the lives of Latino gay men, making it impossible for many to put their intentions into action to reduce risk in their sexual practice. Diaz argues that the interrelated effects of machismo, homophobia, family loyalty, sexual silence, poverty, and racism in the experience of minority Latino populations in the contemporary United States combine to produce a psycho-cultural model that, together with specific psychosexual scripts for regulation of sexual conduct, profoundly limits the possibilities of Latino gay men for self-regulation and risk reduction. His analysis offers a powerful critique of the limitations of dominant cognitive-behavioral theories of behavior change in response to HIV/ AIDS, focusing, in contrast, on the urgent need for culturally appropriate, community based, intervention strategies capable of enabling Latino gay men to transform intentions into action by reinventing sexual scripts free from the damaging effects of intertwined oppressions.

Many of the same issues resonate in chapter 10, "Gendered Scripts and the Sexual Scene: Promoting Sexual Subjects among Brazilian Teenagers," by Vera Paiva. Like Diaz, Paiva seeks to re-think the kinds of intervention strategies that have dominated education and prevention approaches to HIV/AIDS vulnerability, not only in the United States but, through its influence, in countries around the world. Through detailed analysis of the roles of gender and sexuality in the experience of young night school students from impoverished inner-city neighborhoods in São Paulo, she is able to look at the multiple ways structural forces impact upon, and limit the choices available to, boys as well as girls—who find themselves equally trapped in a prison house at once symbolic and material. Rejecting the imposition of North American models of behavior change in favor of the long-standing Latin American tradition of popular education and liberation pedagogy (perhaps most widely associated with the influential work of Paulo Freire, and ironically rediscovered in Brazil only after more than a decade of information-based, cognitive-behavioral intervention programs, and applying this model creatively to the fundamentally new subject matter of gender power and sexual oppression, Paiva, with her colleagues, offers a conceptual framework for the deconstruction and reconstruction of gender relations and sexual experience through a dialogical and dialectical methodology originally pioneered in struggles against illiteracy and class oppression. By focusing on such theoretical and methodological interfaces, Paiva succeeds in highlighting the extent to which individual and collective empowerment are mutually implicated in a broader process of *"concientização"* or "consciousness raising" integral to the constitution of sexual subjects in *all* social and cultural settings.

Finally, in chapter 11, "The Production of Knowledge on Sexuality in the AIDS Era: Some Issues, Opportunities, and Challenges," included as Afterword to the preceding empirical studies, Carlos Cácares assesses some key challenges that have emerged in sex research over recent decades, arguing that, in the wake of the HIV/AIDS pandemic and with the consolidation of agenda linked to the promotion of sexual health and reproductive rights, sexuality has come, more than ever, to constitute a broad, contested field of play. Growing demand for academic and scientific work in this area has transformed institutional, disciplinary, and political boundaries of knowledge production concerning the sexual, and has involved an increasingly complex array of social actors. The authority of psychologists and biomedical specialists has increasingly been contested not only by sociologists and anthropologists but by activists for women's rights and women's health, for alternative sexualities, for environmental justice, and for abortion rights, and by AIDS activists, lawyers and politicians, health care providers, religious leaders, and journalists—as much in the industrialized countries as in the post-colonial developing world. Arguing strongly for a notion of positioned knowledges, as opposed to a myth of neutral or objective science, Cáceres suggests that hermeneutic and epistemological concerns increasingly become ethical and political questions. Researchers reposition themselves as political actors "with specific stakes in a contested field"—and, recognizing this, the true enormity of the efforts ultimately needed to change the oppressive realities not only of the past but of the present begins to become apparent.

Of course, the texts brought together in this volume are but a small contribution to a much broader collective project. Situated, however, at the point of intersection of such diverse currents, and consistently focused on the need to critically interpret the world to change it, these studies offer insight into the kinds of analysis and action that are urgently needed. While addressing a range of issues and positioned in many different ways, they are uncompromising in their desire to link theory to practice and to deconstruct the sorts of hierarchies and hegemonies that have long operated within the production and re-production of sexual knowledges. Ultimately, it is only through such committed work that we can hope to reinvent the politics of gender, sexuality, and power in the future—to create a world in which we can all be the subjects of our own sexualities, and the agents of our own sexual and sexualized histories.

Notes

1. The signs of this boom vary from one setting to the next. At the most obvious level, they include the rapid growth of publications related to almost all aspects of sexuality. More specifically, there is the growing interest of funding agencies. In the United States, for example, a number of prominent foundations, including the Ford Foundation, John D. and Catherine T. Mac-Arthur Foundation, and Rockefeller Foundation, came together in the early 1990s to fund an "assessment" of the state of the art in the field of sexuality research (Di Mauro, 1995, 1997); following this assessment, a new fellowship program was established at the Social Science Research Council to fund graduate student and postdoctoral research on sexuality in the U.S. While there have been highly publicized debates about the role of government funding (or its lack [Laumann, Gagnon, and Michael, 1994]), high-profile national surveys of sexual behavior have been carried out in many major Western countries, including the U.S., Britain, and France. Even in the U.S. federal agencies such as the National Institutes of Health have increasingly provided support for health-related research on sexual behavior, first in the context of HIV/AIDS (particularly at the National Institute of Mental Health), but increasingly in relation to broader demographic and population issues (at, for example, the National Institute of Child Health and Development). Internationally, these trends are also observable, particularly in relation to work on sexuality sponsored by the World Health Organization through its Global Programme on AIDS (WHO/GPA) and through its Programme on Human Reproduction (WHO/HRP), as well as in a number of programs sponsored by bilateral donors such as the United States Agency for International Development (Parker, 1997).

2. On the history of sexology and scientific research on sexuality, see for example the discussions in Foucault, 1978; Irvine, 1990; Parker and Gagnon, 1995; Robinson, 1976; and Weeks, 1985, 1986. On an alternative current in sexuality research, see also the articles republished in Parker and Aggleton, 1999.

3. In addition to this traditional focus on behavioral research in the field of public health, it is important that the HIV/AIDS epidemic first emerged

in the U.S. during the 1980s, at the height of the "Reagan revolution" in American politics. Within this context, research focusing on individual psychology was more politically and ideologically acceptable than were more sociological approaches. Much the same political climate was also present in Great Britain—where Prime Minister Margaret Thatcher looked suspiciously upon social science research generally—as well as in many of the countries where social and behavioral research on HIV/AIDS was first initiated. Indeed, it is quite striking that in Australia, one of the few industrialized democracies with a more progressive political climate during this period, a very different approach to social research on HIV/AIDS emerged early in the epidemic (see for example the discussions in Kirp and Bayer, 1992; see also Kippax, Connell, Dowsett, and Crawford, 1993; Dowsett, 1996). A similar interaction between political climate or context and the conduct of research can of course be seen in relation to biomedical investigation; for a detailed and nuanced account of the relations between social and political context and biomedical AIDS research, see in particular Epstein, 1996.

4. It is perhaps not surprising that much of this work first emerged in cross-cultural research, and in the analysis of non-Western settings where the biomedical categories of epidemiological analysis failed to be fully applicable. Increasingly, however, cultural analysis has also been developed in specific sexual cultures or subcultures in the industrialized West, offering important new insights even in settings where extensive behavioral research had already been carried out.

References

Aggleton, P. (ed.). (1996a). *Bisexualities and AIDS: International Perspectives*. London: Taylor and Francis.

———. (1996b). "Global Priorities for HIV/AIDS Intervention Research." *International Journal of STD and AIDS*, 7(suppl 2).

———. (ed.). (1998). *Men Who Sell Sex: International Perspectives on Male Prostitution and HIV/AIDS*. London: UCL Press, and Philadelphia: Temple Press.

Aggleton, P., and Coates, T. (1995). "Social, Cultural, and Political Aspects." *AIDS*, 9(suppl A): S237–38.

Ajzen, I., and Fishbein, M. (1980). *Understanding Attitudes and Predicting Behavior*. Englewood Cliffs, NJ: Prentice-Hall.

Alonso, A. M., and Koreck, M. T. (1989). "Silences: 'Hispanics,' AIDS, and Sexual Practices." *Differences: A Journal of Feminist Cultural Studies*, 1: 101–24.

Altman, D. (1994). *Power and Community: Organizational and Cultural Responses to AIDS*. London: Taylor and Francis.

Bancroft, J. (ed.). (1997). *Researching Sexual Behavior: Methodological Issues*. Bloomington: Indiana University Press.

Bandura, A. (1977). *Social Learning Theory*. Englewood Cliffs, NJ: Prentice-Hall.

Becker, M., and Joseph, J. K. (1988). "AIDS and Behavioral Change to Reduce Risk: A Review." *American Journal of Public Health*, 78:394–410.

Bishop, R., and Robinson, L. S. (1998). *Night Market: Sexual Cultures and the Thai Economic Miracle*. New York and London: Routledge.

Butler, J. (1990). *Gender Trouble: Feminism and the Subversion of Identity*. New York and London: Routledge.

Carballo, M., Cleland, J., Caraël, M., and Albrecht, G. (1989). "A Cross-National Study of Patterns of Sexual Behavior." *The Journal of Sex Research*, 26:287–99.

Chouinard, A., and Albert, J. (eds.). (1989). *Human Sexuality: Research Perspectives in a World Facing AIDS*. Ottawa: International Development Research Centre.

Cleland, J., and Ferry, B. (eds.). (1995). *Sexual Behaviour and AIDS in the Developing World*. London: Taylor and Francis.

Cohen, M. (1991). "Changing to Safer Sex: Personality, Logic, and Habit." In Aggleton, P., Hart, G., and Davies, P., (eds.), *AIDS: Responses, Interventions and Care*, 19–42. London: Falmer Press.

Corrêa, S. (1994). *Population and Reproductive Rights: Feminist Perspectives from the South*. London: Zed Books.

Daniel, H., and Parker, R. G. (1993). *Sexuality, Politics, and AIDS in Brazil*. London: Falmer Press.

de Zalduondo, B. O. (1991). "Prostitution Viewed Cross-Culturally: Toward Recontextualizing Sex Work in AIDS Intervention Research." *The Journal of Sex Research*, 33:223–48.

de Zalduondo, B. O., and Bernard, J. M. (1995). "Meanings and Consequences of Sexual-Economic Exchange: Gender, Poverty, and Sexual Risk Behavior in Urban Haiti." In Parker, R. G., and Gagnon, J., (eds.), *Conceiving Sexuality: Approaches to Sex Research in a Postmodern World*, 157–80. New York and London: Routledge.

Di Mauro, D. (1995). *Sexuality Research in the United States: An Assessment of the Social and Behavioral Sciences*. New York: Social Science Research Council.

———. (1997). "Sexuality Research in the United States." In Bancroft, J. (ed.), *Researching Sexual Behavior: Methodological Issues*, 3–8. Bloomington: Indiana University Press.

Dowsett, G. W. (1996). *Practicing Desire: Homosexual Sex in the Era of AIDS*. Stanford: Stanford University Press.

Epstein, S. (1996). *Impure Science: AIDS, Activism, and the Politics of Knowledge*. Berkeley and Los Angeles: University of California Press.

Farmer, P., Connors, M., and Simmons, J. (eds.). (1996). *Women, Poverty, and AIDS: Sex, Drugs, and Structural Violence*. Monroe, Maine: Common Courage Press.

Foucault, M. (1978). *The History of Sexuality*, Vol. 1, *An Introduction*. New York: Pantheon.

Garber, M. (1992). *Vested Interests: Cross-Dressing and Cultural Anxiety*. New York: Routledge.

Geertz, C. (1983). *Local Knowledge*. New York: Basic Books.

Ginsberg, F., and Rapp, R. (eds.). (1995). *Conceiving the New World Order: The Global Politics of Reproduction*. Berkeley and Los Angeles: University of California Press.

Haraway, D. (1991). *Simians, Cyborgs, and Women: The Reinvention of Nature*. New York and London: Routledge.

Harvey, D. (1990). *The Condition of Postmodernity*. Cambridge, MA, and Oxford: Blackwell.

Heise, L. (1995). "Violence, Sexuality, and Women's Lives." In Parker, R. G., and Gagnon, J., (eds.). *Conceiving Sexuality: Approaches to Sex Research in a Postmodern World*, 109–34. New York and London: Routledge.

Herdt, G. (1997). *Same Sex, Different Cultures: Gays and Lesbians Across Cultures*. Boulder and Oxford: Westview Press.

———. (ed.). (1993). *Third Sex, Third Gender: Beyond Sexual Dimorphism in Culture and History*. New York: Zone Books.

Herdt G., and Lindenbaum, S. (eds.). (1992). *The Time of AIDS: Social Analysis, Theory and Method*. Newbury Park: Sage Publications.

Hyam, R. (1990). *Empire and Sexuality: The British Experience*. Manchester: Manchester University Press.

Irvine, J. (1990). *Disorders of Desire*. Philadelphia: Temple University Press.

Kippix, S., Connell, R. W., Dowsett, G. W., and Crawford, J. (1993). *Sustaining Safe Sex: Gay Communities Respond to AIDS*. London: Taylor and Francis.

Kippax, S., and Crawford, J. (1993). "Flaws in the Theory of Reasoned Action." In Terry, D. J., Gallois, C., and McCamish, M. M., (eds.), *Theory of Reasoned Action: Its Applications to AIDS-Preventive Behaviour*, 253–69. London: Pergamon.

Kirp, D., and Bayer, R. (eds.). (1992). *AIDS in the Industrialized Democracies*. New Brunswick: Rutgers University Press.

Kulick, D. (1998). *Travesti: Sex, Gender and Culture among Brazilian Transgendered Prostitutes*. Chicago: University of Chicago Press.

Lancaster, R. N. (1992). *Life is Hard: Machismo, Danger, and the Intimacy of Power in Nicaragua*. Berkeley and Los Angeles: University of California Press.

———. (1995). " 'That We Should All Turn Queer?': Homosexual Stigma in the Making of Manhood and the Breaking of a Revolution in Nicaragua." In Parker, R. G., and Gagnon, J., (eds.), *Conceiving Sexuality: Approaches to Sex Research in a Postmodern World*, 135–56. New York and London: Routledge.

———. (1997). "Sexual Positions: Caveats and Second Thoughts on 'Categories'" *The Americas*, 54 (1 July): 1–16.

Lancaster, R. N., and di Leonardo, M. (eds.). (1997). *The Gender/Sexuality Reader: Culture, History, Political Economy*. New York and London: Routledge.

Laumann, E., Gagnon, J., and Michael, R. (1994). "A Political History of the National Sex Survey of Adults." *Family Planning Perspectives*, 26: 34–38.

Manderson, L., and Jolly, M. (eds.). (1997). *Sites of Desire, Economies of Pleasure: Sexualities in Asia and the Pacific*. Chicago: University of Chicago Press.

Nanda, S. (1985). "The Hijras of India: Cultural and Individual Dimensions of an Institutionalized Third Gender Role." *Journal of Homosexuality*, 11 (3/4):35–54.

Parker, R. G. (1989). "Youth, Identity, and Homosexuality: The Changing Shape of Sexual Life in Brazil." *Journal of Homosexuality*, 17 (3/4): 267–87.

———. (1991). *Bodies, Pleasures, and Passions: Sexual Culture in Contemporary Brazil*. Boston: Beacon Press.

———. (1994). "Sexual Cultures, HIV Transmission, and AIDS Prevention." *AIDS*, 8(suppl):S309–14.

———. (1995). "Behavior in Latin American Men: Implications for HIV/AIDS Interventions." *International Journal of STD and AIDS*, 7(suppl 2):62–65.

———. (1996). "Empowerment, Community Mobilization, and Social Change in the Face of HIV/AIDS." *AIDS*, 10(suppl 3):S27–S31.

———. (1997). "International Perspectives on Sexuality Research." In Bancroft, J. (ed.), *Researching Sexual Behavior: Methodological Issues*, 9–22. Bloomington: Indiana University Press.

———. (1999). *Beneath the Equator: Cultures of Desire, Male Homosexuality, and Emerging Gay Communities in Brazil*. New York and London: Routledge.

Parker, R. G., and Aggleton, P. (eds.). (1999). *Culture, Society, and Sexuality: A Reader*. London: UCL Press.

Parker, R. G., and Barbosa, R. M. (eds.). (1996). *Sexualidades Brasileiras*. Rio de Janeiro: Relume-Dumará.

Parker, R. G., and Carballo, M. (1990). "Qualitative Research on Homosexual and Bisexual Behavior Relevant to HIV/AIDS." *The Journal of Sex Research*, 27(4):497–525.

Parker, R. G., and Easton, D. (1998). "Sexuality, Culture, and Political Economy: Recent Developments in Anthropological and Cross-Cultural Sex Research." *Annual Review of Sex Research*, 9:1–19.

Parker, R. G., and Gagnon, J. (eds.). (1995). *Conceiving Sexuality: Approaches to Sex Research in a Postmodern World*. New York and London: Routledge.

Parker, R. G., Herdt, G., and Carballo, M. (1991). "Sexual Culture, HIV Transmission, and AIDS Research." *The Journal of Sex Research*, 28:77–98.

Parker, R. G., and Terto Jr., V. (eds.). (1998). *Entre Homens: Homossexualidade e AIDS no Brasil*. Rio de Janeiro: ABIA.

Patton, C. (1990). *Inventing AIDS*. New York and London: Routledge.

Petchesky, R., and Judd, K. (eds.). (1998). *Negotiating Reproductive Rights: Women's Perspectives across Countries and Cultures*. London: Zed Books.

Prieur, A. (1998). *Mema's House, Mexico City: On Transvestites, Queens, and Machos*. Chicago and London: University of Chicago Press.

Rao Gupta, G., and Weiss, E. (1995). "Women's Lives and Sex: Implications for AIDS Prevention." In Parker, R. G., and Gagnon, J., (eds.), *Conceiving Sexuality: Approaches to Sex Research in a Postmodern World*, 259–70. New York and London: Routledge.

Robinson, P. (1976). *The Modernization of Sex*. New York: Harper and Row.

Rubin, G. (1975). "The Traffic in Women: Notes on the 'Political Economy' of Sex." In Reiter, R. (ed.), *Toward an Anthropology of Women*. New York: Monthly Review Press.

———. (1984). "Thinking Sex: Notes for a Radical Theory of the Politics of Sexuality." In Vance, C. S. (ed.), *Pleasure and Danger: Exploring Female Sexuality*, 267–319. London: Routledge and Kegan Paul.

Scott, J. (1986). "Gender as a Useful Category of Historical Analysis." *American Historical Review*, 91, no. 5.

Singer, M. (ed.). (1998). *The Political Economy of AIDS*. Amityville, NY: Baywood Publishing Company.

Snitow, A., Stansell, C., and Thompson, S. (eds.). (1983). *Powers of Desire*. New York: Monthly Review Press.

Stein, Z. (1990). "HIV Prevention: The Need for Methods Women Can Use." *American Journal of Public Health*, 80:460–62.

Stoler, A. L. (1995). *Race and the Education of Desire: Foucault's History of Sexuality and the Colonial Order of Things*. Durham: Duke University Press.

Sweat, M. D., and Dennison, J. A. (1995). "Reducing HIV Incidence in Developing Countries with Structural and Environmental Interventions." *AIDS*, 9(suppl A):S251–57.

Treichler, P. (1992). "AIDS and the Cultural Construction of Reality." In Herdt, G., and Lindenbaum, S., (eds.), *The Time of AIDS: Social Analysis, Theory, and Method*, 65–100. Newbury Park, CA: Sage.

Turner, C. F., Miller, H. G., and Moses, L. E. (eds.). (1989). *AIDS: Sexual*

Behavior and Intravenous Drug Use. Washington, DC: National Academy Press.

———. (1990). *AIDS: The Second Decade*. Washington, DC: National Academy Press.

Vance, C. S. (1991). "Anthropology Rediscovers Sexuality: A Theoretical Comment." *Sociological and Scientific Medicine* 33(8):875–84.

Vance, C. S. (ed.). (1984). *Pleasure and Danger: Exploring Female Sexuality*. New York: Routledge and Kegan Paul.

Watney, S. (1990). "Safer Sex as Community Practice." In Aggleton, P., Hart, G., and Davies, P., (eds.), *AIDS: Individual, Cultural, and Policy Dimensions*, 19–35. London: Falmer Press.

———. (1994). *Practices of Freedom: Selected Writings on HIV/AIDS*. Durham: Duke University Press.

Weeks, J. (1985). *Sexuality and its Discontents: Meanings, Myths, and Modern Sexualities*. London: Routledge and Kegan Paul.

———. (1986). *Sexuality*. London: Tavistock.

Young, R. J. C. (1995). *Colonial Desire: Hybridity in Theory, Culture, and Race*. London and New York: Routledge.

Part One

Bodies, Cultures, and Identities

Chapter One

Bodyplay

Corporeality in a Discursive Silence

Gary W. Dowsett

It is quite dark, the eyes take a while to focus. As the vision clears, he comes into view. Lying naked, facedown on a padded bench surrounded by shoulder-high partitions, he has put his desire "on-line," with a box of condoms and lubricant nearby. A man, also naked, approaches slowly, silently, and reaches out to brush ever so lightly the buttocks of the man on the bench. The slow stroking expands its ambit, covering the body from back of neck to back of knee, focusing its attention on arousing the arousing buttocks. In the dim light, others congregate to watch from the doorway or over the partitions. More glistening eyes come into view. Soon they too are being stroked, more insistently, more confidently.

The man on the couch lifts his head a little and briefly surveys the congregation, notes the erect man at his side, and slowly lowers his head onto folded arms. He raises his buttocks slightly to the touch of his attendant, giving consent. Over the next hour, the man on the bench is fucked by ten men in sequence, always with condoms, always with his head cradled on folded arms, after the first glance never seeking to assess the successors laboring upon him, and only in momentary crescendoes arching backwards to receive more fully his thrusting devotees in their perverse salute to the sun.

Surrounding him, others come and go, aroused, sated, included visually or physically in the performance or merely satisfied to bear witness to yet another re-presentation of "the internalized phallic male as an infinitely loved object of sacrifice" (Bersani, 1988, 222).

———

For me there is a certain terror, even a certain sense of betrayal, in describing the above events. Permission to gaze upon this sex event was granted to the men present, not to you as readers. This was no Masters and Johnson laboratory, with clinical setting and white coats absolving scientists from their desire. Nor does my reservation derive from ethical issues about informed consent in sexuality research, even if participant observation poses its own ethical problems. But there is still a sense in which this sex event, selectively available to men throughout history, and ever changing in its succeeding representations, should be only for the initiated, for those male bodies pursuing what we have only recently called *homosexuality*.

My anxiety comes also from the risk of being misunderstood. How do I convince those who have never witnessed or experienced such an encounter, of its particular logic, its contextualized intentions, its cultural specificities? How does one explain academically what engages men when faced with the "pigpen of pulchritude" (Coe, 1993, 299). These silent events are symphonies in erotics, performed in the suspension of time that sex often engenders—a suspension described better by poets and novelists than by sex researchers.

This event is part of the picture that fills what has been described as Foucault's empty frame of sexuality (Connell and Dowsett, 1993); this event is a *fact* in the intersection of discourses that construct sexuality. Yet I want to distance such events from this intersection, for it always casts them as quotient or product, always assimilates them within power. I am not reiterating some gay liberation trope here; this is not some rehash of John Rechy's "sexual outlaws" (1977); nor am I attempting to frame such sex acts as refusal (Weeks, 1985) or realignment (Bristow, 1989). After all, no man in the sex event described had his mind on challenging the sexual or social order. But I want to avoid the trap that renders such events as always already inscribed within Foucault's deployment of sexuality, and in this sense necessarily defeated at their moment of origin.

Such sex events offer us a challenge: to re-think such events as "big bang" moments, moments of creation, moments where sexuality comes into being not merely in an intersection of discourses pinpointing subjectivity like a butterfly in a museum display case, but where sexuality itself is *constructed* (not "represented") by bodies-in-sex. To grasp this potentiality, we need to move beyond the textuality of discourse toward the texturality of the body—for the mime in which bodies-in-sex collectively make sensation and re-make meaning actually drowns out the larger, more structural din of sexuality, as we know it post-Foucault. It might be that sexuality has become an emperor without clothes, and we are forced again to contemplate a naked body. I want to contemplate that body not simply as the *incorporation* of sexuality, but as a body operating sexually in a *discursive silence*. This discursive silence is like a black hole, not empty but full of density, itself offering a discrete corporeality.

The role of erotics in sex events is immediately intelligible to anyone present, yet rarely are words spoken; such lore is not handed down in that kind of oral tradition. Completing a satisfying collective sexual encounter without speech requires not only the learned sexual skill of gay men in recognising their own desire in each other and matching it, but also on the deeply relational character of such engagements. In this concatenation of the relational and the embodied may be found something disturbingly new about sexuality.

I want first to look at two elements in relation to the body: sexual practice, and the relations of sex. And I shall do this by presenting a brief life history of a man I interviewed as part of my ongoing ethnographic investigation of Australian gay men's sexuality in the era of HIV/AIDS (Dowsett, 1996). Second, I want to explore the relationality of gay sex, with a view to discussing the sexual construction of sociality as my third point.

The Body in Sex

Harry Wight learned about sex with boys at a young age. Harry had a regular "wankette" with another boy after school and on Saturday mornings before and after swimming lessons; they would always strip naked at the local changing room. Other boys and similar events followed, mutual masturbation mainly, and eventually an initiation in anal sex—with an older boy, although it was Harry who did the inserting.

Many other men I have interviewed over the last ten years of research reported similar childhood experiences—regular sex games with neighbors, with schoolmates, sometimes with older men. The boys taught each other about erections and the orifices they might

penetrate, about the pleasures of arousal, and inevitably about ejaculation. Most learned sex acts with peers; occasionally older youths
or siblings were involved. Some reported learning from schoolmates
of places (called in Australia "beats," and usually public parks or toilet
blocks) to find sex with grown men and with other boys. Such sex play
was not furtive, but was carried on away from the gaze of parents and
other adults. It was also a very sociable activity, collectively pursued,
yet free from the preponderant discursive definition to which sexuality
is often prone. In this sense, such sexual exploration occurred in social
lacunae in which the operation of general prohibitive and regulatory
discourses on sex was imperfect and patchy in penetration. Its success,
if any, lay in producing secrecy, not celibacy.

Harry had already had considerable sexual experience with other
boys when he first heard the word "poofter". "What's a poofter?" he
naively asked a schoolmate on the bus one day. As the other boy
alighted, he answered for all to hear, "Someone who pisses up ya'
bum and it feels great!" Even more significant as countervailing narrative, however, was the pleasure being experienced in, on, or through
the bodies of other boys. These bodies-in-sex, wilfully oblivious to
definition and denial, were producing a collective sexual culture long
before any of the boys heard of poofters, buggers, sodomites, gay
men, Oscar Wilde—or Michel Foucault. In their example, we have
to tackle seriously the formative contribution of the body's early experiences in sex—of first pain and first pleasure, fearful first ejaculation, mutual manipulations of like bodies, and the unique pleasures
of the male prostate—the formative contribution, indeed, of penetration first experienced in discursive silence, in which no sheepish,
oblique, or ill-defined discourse on sodomy counters the unnamed
and, at that time, unnamable bodily sensations of being fucked.

We must take seriously also the contribution of these skilling and
satisfying activities in producing the sexually proficient youths and
men who later encounter the deployment of sexuality in, as Foucault
puts it, a more exacting and incisive form. Harry, for instance, proved
a less than willing subject for sexuality. In early adolescence, he met
his future wife and homosex stopped for a few years. After a while,
however, this changed. His girlfriend would come to dinner each Sunday and they would have sex afterwards—but that was Sunday. On
Thursdays, Harry went to college, and at age eighteen, the now-
engaged young man, on his way to class one evening, stopped in a

public toilet at a railway station: "Anyway, I was standing there having a leak and this guy came in. And all of a sudden it just kinda clicked. And he stood there and I stood there and I remembered what I used to do before. And he said to me: 'Do you want to?' and I'd cracked a fat [got an erection], and he said: 'Do you want me to do something about it?' And I said: 'No, I don't.' I just sucked him . . ."

About a month later in the same beat, Harry accepted an invitation to a married man's empty home, again missing class. This time Harry fucked the guy; it was Harry's first fully successful anal penetration. Needless to say, Harry failed college that year, as his new-found thrill became a regular pastime. He would meet the same man regularly, and his partner taught him the sexual ropes—kissing, oral sex, anal sex. Eventually Harry let the guy fuck him, but it hurt and Harry remained an insertive partner after that.

Harry had sex with other men in that beat and, soon, in others. He worked in the central business district, and found other toilets at railway stations and in parks to visit en route to and from his job and during lunch hour. Thus he came to know of a significant sexual network throughout the city and its suburbs—a pleasure map by which he navigated through his day.

Some men in my research filled their days by meandering through these possibilities. Many accounts in the study tell of men pursuing beat sex avidly, reporting repeated encounters with multiple partners. As one described it: "I can remember coming from [a suburb] to Sydney and calling in at a series of beats on the way and getting screwed eight times, and just loving that. This was the pre-safe-sex days . . . I can still remember, part of the deliciousness of it was the feeling of cum dripping out of my arse and the slipperiness of my cheeks moving past each other as lubrication." There is more than a hint of "trespass" here, of walking the streets bearing silent witness to male-to-male sexual transgression—lots of it, and in public places. Having another man's semen inside one's rectum is an insistent motif in much gay poetry and fiction, and its forfeiture a serious issue to deal with in HIV prevention. And it would appear that women are not the only ones with worries about wet patches.

Harry's success, and the readily available beat partners, speak of an active sexuality where a man's penetrability, far from providing the comfortable analogue of the passive vagina (or, once upon a time, allowing science its "invert"), demands that we engage the possibility of sexual encounters where both partners must be regarded as phallic. We are reminded not to mistake the penis for the phallus; these sexual interests cannot be reduced to men's capacity for ready erection and quick orgasm. What is important is the reciprocal nature of the encounters, the easy exchange of pleasure rather than its "taking," the desiring anus, and the active fingers, hands, mouths, penises, lips, tongues, semen, and sweat involved. There is no denying the physicality; it is *bodies* in sex that are central here, and no discursive incursion on the beastly nature of sodomy, fellatio, anilingus, or fist- and finger-fucking achieves its mark against the lure of the body-in-sex.

There is undoubtedly a strong bodily pull in this "toilet tango," as Oscar Moore (1991) exalts it; the fantasizing body displays or enjoins a "disembodied" yet, at the same time, palpably corporeal penis in the "glory hole" or under the partition; eager anonymous anuses are read like braille in the darkness. Sex of such caliber is not without other dimensions; the sexual possibilities provided by beats mean that they become not only sites of promise of unending pleasure, but also signifiers of, and spaces for, exploring the elsewhere unattainable or unavailable—of pursuing the fantastic. In this regard, homosexually active men have created and developed worldwide sexual cultures that can be explored anywhere, in any language—yet without words— and with increasing concentration as global urbanization expands. Thus our cities are made sexually.

But back to Harry, who knew little of this global wonder. In marriage, he and his wife soon lost the ardor of their youth, and he turned his sexual attentions increasingly toward men. Beat sex continued uninterrupted during the decade of the marriage. Harry occasionally ventured out to the odd social event with other homosexual men. He went to his first inner-suburban gay dance—a "smorgasbord," he called it in retrospect—but experienced no sense of connectedness to what he saw there. One or two of his sex partners became his friends. He met gay couples, and he started an affair with another married man, but quickly finished it when it became a bit "serious." Beat sex was his mainstay.

As Harry's experience shows, the beats provide for a slow development of social relations, beyond sex itself, among homosexually active men—nascent relationships, stop-start affairs, new friendships—and can be places to meet others and just talk. What is important in this is the sociality developing out of sex. This layering of meaning and potential is hardly captured by those terms we so often use for such sex acts in our behavioral surveys and HIV/AIDS safe-sex monitoring: "casual," "anonymous," "impersonal." This activity is anything but casual; it requires familiarity with the choreography of sexual pursuit and action, and the patience and dedication of a champion. It is never anonymous; are lovers less lovers for their silence? There is nothing impersonal in achieving mutuality in the concupiscent collision of desiring bodies.

Such sociality can build, transform. Harry reported the following event as his first truly wonderful sexual experience. He met a near-naked man in a park:

H: And I really think that was the first time I ever made *love* to a man.

GD: Really, was it just straight sex until that moment?

H: It was all sex, straight raw sex up until then. He said: "Would you like to come with me?" and I said: "Would I ever!" He took me up into the bushes type thing in the car, and he made love.

GD: What's the difference?

H: John [his partner] and I do it. We do it—sometimes we just screw, just fuck, and then other times we just make love.

GD: Can you give some words to describe it? I don't mean describe it like in a sentence, but just actually words, like sensual, touch.

H: A bit of touch, a bit of—I mean [pause] it probably might just happen in the time of your life when you most need it . . .

GD: With two people at the same moment?

H: Yes. Can you relate to what I'm talking about?

GD: Oh yes, absolutely. I just wanted you to spell it out.

H: [laughter] I mean, this guy was—although I stripped off with K—— earlier on when I was a kid, and I probably stripped off with all of them, this bloke *undressed* me. There was no quick grab hold of your cock and wank it and get your mouth around it. There was feeling to it. There was touching to it. And did I get in the shit when I got home, 'cause I was probably there for about three hours. And he taught me how to kiss. He taught me how to put your tongue out, and not leave it there, which annoys me . . . Just took his time with me.

GD: The magic moment, eh?

H: It doesn't happen often.

This moment initiated a process of transformation in Harry. It illuminated the possibilities in male-to-male sex beyond orgasm, beyond one level of reciprocity. Something more, something indefinable, glimmered for him in this short affair that got "serious." Soon that glimmer came sharply into view in the relationship he developed with John.

Harry had a rule about casual sex partners at that time; he never saw the same person more than twice. This decision was designed to protect himself from the emotional connection he had realized was possible, as well as to protect his marriage, and reveals again the relational complexity of so-called "impersonal" homosex events. Harry met John in a beat and after having sex, he and John *talked*! Talking can be so dangerous; it jeopardizes a fragile anonymity, it beckons intimacy. The two men met again after work for a drink. They discovered that their situations were similar: both married with kids, sexually interested in men, "average blokes" (as Harry called them), and regular beat users. In penetrative sex, one preferred to be receptive, the other to insert. The major difference between them was the state of their sexual identities. John's wife had known he was homosexual when they married. Harry's had known nothing of his sexual interests.

Eventually, the men's growing sense of connectedness developed into a strong emotional and sexual relationship. John's wife apparently knew about it, and finally told friends that he intended to leave her. This pushed Harry into the decision he had so far put off. His wife had by then realized he was homosexual. After a painful breakup, Harry and John began living together; they had been together for ten years when I met them.

Harry's story reveals the centrality of the body, its explorations, and its sensations to the construction of a life—to patterns of living, balance of preoccupations, decisions, and directions. The story also illuminates the recognition of the self in the body—that *being* Harry is measured in the body. When Harry's body engaged other men, it was that body's sensations and experience that led him. It was the searing pain in his anus that caused him subsequently to forgo being penetrated. It was his tongue that was taught not to hang out, his skin that was always bared, gaining further arousal and pleasure from the sight of others' skin. It was his "cracking a fat" that reminded him of pleasures foregone during his courting days. Finally, it was the experience of his whole body making love in the bushes that taught him there was more to men than "raw sex."

This is a story of *embodied* intensities and an increasing determination to pleasure, in a working-class man without recourse to gay liberation tropés or complex theories of sexuality. In the light of this active pursuit of homosex, we cannot simply regard Harry's body as passively awaiting the inscription of the social. Whatever intrusions discourses made upon his sex life, they never persuaded Harry to give it up. At each point, his embodied engagement with homosex more than countered any specific anti-homosexual discourse that came his way. It is clear the physical human body is actively in play here, but not as some pre-social body with asocial capacities awaiting social inscription. Just as there is no longer room for a biology, a physical science of the body, separate from the social body, so a social theory of the body that neglects its biology remains flawed. The body itself teaches and inscribes.

There is another aspect to Harry's tale—the markedly delayed development of more intense relational aspects of his homosexuality. This delay allows us analytically to join the body and its sex practices, mark them off from relationality, and focus on the body itself. But relationality, which eventually did come, quickly confirmed a fully fleshed-out life for Harry as a gay man. The developing relational intensities of Harry's long homosexual experimentation were evident to himself. That relational potential finally bloomed with John, yet the physicality of their long relationship remained; when I interviewed Harry, they still fucked like bunnies often, specializing in threesomes with married men regularly picked up at the local beat. The sexual construction of their relationship did not overshadow other aspects of their life together, but was central to its organization.

Relationality

A different account of sexuality emerges among a more recent generation of men for which "gay" already existed, but which still demonstrates the formative action of the body-in-sex, this time deeply embedded within a relationality that encodes sensation. This account must reinsert the relational into an investigation of sex as embodied yet not lose the body-in-sex inside relationality.

I recently read the posthumously published, semi-autobiographical

Holding the Man by Timothy Conigrave (1995). Conigrave was an Australian actor, playwright, gay activist, and HIV/AIDS educator. His bestselling book documents his fifteen-year relationship with his lover John, ending just after John's death from AIDS—a year before Conigrave's own, also from AIDS, late in 1994.

As fifteen-year-old boys at a Catholic high school starting the relationship of their lives, Tim and John were fearless in pursuing sex. Their first fuck occurred after a few dates and lots of intense kissing. On a school retreat together:

John and I were lying head to toe on my bed. It was nice being close to him like this. I could feel the warmth radiating from him. John took hold of my feet, held them close to his cheeks and starting kissing them gently.

"What are you doing?" I whispered, alarmed.

"I don't know. I just want to."

My feet were alive with his soft stroking and gentle kissing. "You'd better stop, I'm cracking a fat."

"Good, so am I," John said seductively.

"What are you two up to? A bit of foot fetish, John?" Joe [a schoolmate] was watching us. He suggested we all sleep on the floor. John and I could lie together without looking sus [suspicious], so we all agreed. As we hauled the mattresses off the bed, Biscuit [another schoolmate] winked. "Never know what might happen."

Among the mattresses, pillows, and throw-cushions, we lay like a sheik's wives in a harem. In the darkness Biscuit and Joe whispered and giggled. John and I were nuzzling noses. He smelt sweet.

Lips caressing lips. Exploring. Our lips slightly parted, exchanging breath. Hands slipping into each other's sleeping-bags. His warm body in cotton PJs [pajamas]. Running my hand up his spine, feeling the muscles in his back. His hand going in under my pajama shirt. Skin of his hand against the skin of my back. My hand slipped into his pants and stroked his downy bum, pulling his hips closer to mine. I wanted to reach round to the front and hold his sex but was scared that it might spin him out. I moved my hand to his stomach and slowly worked it down to play with his bush of pubes, occasionally brushing his erection.

His eyes were shut and his breathing was getting faster. I took hold of his cock in one hand and his cool balls in the other. He started to groan gently in my ear. He was coming in my hand.

He took my cock and held it against his body, undoing his pyjamas. I pumped it against his belly until I came on his stomach. He touched my semen. "Wow." He smeared it over his chest and stomach. "Can you touch me again?"

I took hold of his cock, which was still hard. He started pumping my hand until his body arched and he came again. Still puffing, he hugged me and whispered, "I love you."

We drifted off to sleep, deep, blissful, complete. Through the night we would wake and start kissing, fondling, tugging and coming again. We were two suns, exchanging atmospheres, drawn into each other, spiralling into each other.

I woke in a patch of early morning sun. In front of me was the angelic face of John asleep, almost smiling, his eyelashes against his cheeks. *My boyfriend. And last night we made love for the first time.* (Conigrave, 1995, 92–93, original emphasis)

These early sexual moments between Tim and John are reminders of the impossibility of dissolving the link between relationality and embodiment. Rather as the parents of these two boys tried to separate them, we in sex research struggle to tear apart sex practices and sexual relations, embodiment and relationality. Tim and John's very pursuit of relationally-laden sex and a sexually laden relationship laughs at such attempts.

As Tim's and John's bodies collide, at various times, through the first part of the book, they do so in the most improbable contexts, exemplifying a certain sexual perversity of boys, a willingness to have a feel, to grope in a group, to touch up a tush, to flash and fondle in the showers, to play pocket billiards with each other. They were not yet gay, but they were "boyfriends," and their schoolmates sensed something special going on, even colluding in supporting the relationship in the confines of the school.

Tim and John were constrained by unspecified discourses that prohibited sex and contrived to characterize sexual relations between males in a certain way. They were successful citizens in their high school, John a football captain and prefect, Tim a celebrated actor. Both were also extraordinarily beautiful. Whose bodies, whose desires, might this engage? The Jesuit fathers were therefore concerned about the boys' closeness; the parents at first thought them good for each other, but grew hostile when the sexual nature of the relationship became obvious. But something propelled these two boys toward sex, overwhelming the opposition in skirmishes that lasted throughout their lives, but which, from the beginning, they usually won.

Harry Wight had the same sort of sex play with his peers, if without the same early relational intensity, a generation earlier. It was this cross-generational correspondence in sexual exploration that convinced me these are not minority experiences; rather, in varying degrees and at different times, sexual exchanges between boys can emerge as a significant culture, a widely acknowledged collective experience, witnessed and facilitated, much as their schoolmates willingly assisted John and Tim. These experiences are shared in a variety of ways with other boys—at the level of rumor, near misses, stories, wayward acts, and, for some, sustained practice.

What Tim and John's story also reveals is that the discursive silence in which they explored the potential of their bodies-in-sex was even more silent on the relational possibilities they pursued. Just as Harry, in that moment of revelation, "made love" and recognized something else available in and to men, Tim and John with no help discovered— invented—their relationship, only later seeking gay life to contextualize it, to give it shape and firmer definition. The discursive silence on male relationality that they experienced was filled also by their bodies; there can be no separation of mind and body, emotion and sensation, here.

Sociality

The sexual activities so far described are not pursuits of sexual identity. Neither are they anonymous encounters. Still less are they decontextualized, hormonally charged releases. These engagements are relationally bounded, emotionally grounded, and embodied. It is all in the mix, and to attempt to make sense of sex by ignoring this relationality and merely tallying partner numbers or relationship status, to reify sex acts in essentialist inventories of practices, to relegate the body either to passive receptacle or to a pre-social "nature" awaiting social inscription: these dominant sex-research paradigms are doomed to failure.

This is not a simple argument for a more complex social constructionist perspective on sexuality, in another attempt to move us from the positivist sexological traditions unfortunately reinvigorated with the advent of HIV/AIDS. Rather, it is a plea to move on from the particular preoccupation of social constructionism that renders sexuality as a social product. I want, instead, to argue for a sexual construction of the social.

In this formulation, bodies-in-sex are not awaiting social inscription; rather, our sociality is built through the sexual, and through the enactment of desire—desire not conceived of as lack, as deeply structured need, but as a creation, a "big bang" that produces sexuality. By placing sexuality at the center of the creation of sociality, this conception offers the possibility to rethink the sexual construction of, for example, space, and of identity (rather than its filleted psychic incumbent), of desiring collectivities, and of sexual cultures like those described earlier in this chapter.

There is possibility here for a notion of subjectivity more agentive—and collectively more agentive—available for a politics of sociality seeking to restore sex to a place of constructive relations, in contrast to the increasing confinement of sex to a politics of the improper, the over-determined, the disdained, and the destructive. The separation of bodies-in-sex from the relationality of sexual encounters, even from sexual desire, diminishes our understanding of not only sex but social life. We must place bodies and bodies-in-sex at the heart of sociality not as recipients of inscription but as progenitors of relationality. Such an analysis of sexuality moves us from a sexuality of individual psychologized need toward a mutually creative/created culture of desire.

Foucault was clearly pointing in this direction when, in one of his later interviews, he said: "I think that what most bothers those who are not gay about gayness is the gay lifestyle, not the sex acts themselves. It is the prospect that gays will create as yet unforeseen kinds of relationships that many people cannot tolerate" (quoted in Bersani, 1995, 11). This is correct in positioning the newness of relations among gay men to the fore, but I would suggest that Foucault is also partly mistaken: sex acts between men do themselves significantly trouble many. The epigraph to Leo Bersani's famous essay, "Is the Rectum a Grave?" offers a case in point: "These people have sex twenty to thirty times a night . . . A man comes along and goes from anus to anus and in a single night will act as a mosquito transferring infected cells on his penis. When this is practiced for a year, with a man having three thousand sexual intercourses, one can readily understand this massive epidemic that is currently upon us" (Professor Opendra Narayan, John Hopkins Medical School, quoted in Bersani, 1988, 197).

It is not some new form of relationality that troubles Professor Narayan. If he were to visit a gay bath house, he might indeed witness the enactment of new forms of relationality, in events such as I described earlier, and better understand the epidemic he seeks to stop. But it is clearly the *practice* of homosex that disturbs Professor Narayan—it is the unending buttfucks that get up his nose.

Gay men walking together in Sydney's famous gay precinct, Oxford Street, similarly represent a different relational possibility between men, but it is not their sexual identities that generates anti-gay violence. Such violence is more likely, in the growing gay ghettos of industrialized and Westernized cities, the consequence of the visibility of gay men's relationships. Gay men do confirm very different relational possibilities between men, but they also denote and define certain physical sensations, pleasures foregone or delayed, maybe even remembered. They may distill some inchoate fantasy, unlocking the sexual potential in passivity and the threat to masculinity it inspires. Anti-gay violence is related to the very proximity of men's anuses to their penises. Gay men act as a real and symbolic threat to, and potential for, other men's ever-present penetrability.

I would seek to reassess Foucault's emphasis by positioning sex practices, particularly homosex, centrally in our understanding of sexuality, seeking first deliberately to move the debate from sexuality as identity, "I am," toward sexuality as praxis, "we do". But this maneuver stops short, for it shifts sex and identity only slightly to the side, and fails the challenge of accounting for the collective production of sexual culture and sociality.

In this regard, the question must be asked, is this sociality a mode confined to gay men, to the marginalized who have carved some safe sexy spaces of their own? I think this notion fails to answer the challenge of homosexuality as the pedal point in a homophobic patriarchy as conceived by Eve Kosofsky Sedgwick (1990). If we are to take seriously her universalizing view of homosexuality as *the* constituent of sexuality, rather than as the predominant sexual minority model of identity politics, we can no longer relegate the sex acts of gay men to the margins. These acts may represent, rather, a significant shift at the center; the young Tim and John may already be there.

But we may also have to consider Michel Maffesoli's proposal for reconfiguring a postmodern sociality, one where "what was marginalized during a productive period is diffracted in a multitude of central marginalities" (Maffesoli, 1991, 7). Maffesoli proposes that, in mass society, "processes of condensation are constantly occurring through which more or less ephemeral tribal groupings are organized which cohere on the basis of their own minor values, and which attract and collide with each other in an endless dance, forming themselves into a constellation whose vague boundaries are perfectly fluid. This is the characteristic of postmodern society" (Maffesoli, 1991, 12). Such a shift from the structural proposes that the transcendence we seek in Western sexuality may already be present, but dispersed in ways we have yet to learn. Gay men make this easy for us through their visible sedition.

But gay men in the West form, in their "neo-tribal" sexual activity, a mode of sociality that may also allow us to move beyond what Simon Watney (1986) called the "banality of gender," with its heterosexist preoccupations. Both the bodily pleasures and the reciprocity that Harry explored in sex with men occurred largely within the frame of a life as a heterosexual man—marriage, fatherhood, breadwinner, homeownership, and so on. Harry was one of those "heterosexual" men who have sex with men, so troubling to us in HIV/AIDS work. He was not an example of sexual-identity/sexual-practice dissonance; he did not burden himself with a sexual identity, heterosexual or homosexual, for most of this period of his life (indicating again the limitation of "sexual identity" in sexuality research). Harry Wight did not have a sexual identity; he had no need of one. He only became a *gay man* long after his sexual adventuring with men, when his relationship with John was well established. "Gay" was merely a cultural superimposition that has helped recast the social lives of Harry and John in recent years.

Not only was the binary heterosexual/homosexual irrelevant to Harry, but the development, late in his life, of a more intensive relationality with John contrasts with the easy tropes in gender that privilege, but separate, "gay men" as a special category, allowing the continuing specious category "men" to dominate accounts of sexuality—allowing, that is, continued description of those gay men able to relate well to women as men who can show their emotion, who are in touch with their bodies, and so on. The patronizing tone of such accounts galls; the increasingly simplistic characterization of "men" left in play beyond "gay" would no longer be tolerated in gender theory, particularly by certain forms of feminism, for the category

"women". Yet, unquestioned reliance on that gender binary under-
pins most classic accounts of sexuality in so-called heterosexual epidemics, that dominate HIV/AIDS research.

Why, then, do we continue to reify, in sexuality research, categories
such as "man," "woman," "transgender," "male," "female," "transsex-
ual," "homosexual," "heterosexual," "bisexual"? Why has HIV/AIDS
research failed to learn from the deconstructive scrutiny lavished on
these terms elsewhere—in particular, in cross-cultural research and
post-colonial analyses? We need to look beyond these crude categories, which overlay sexuality with a paradigm of inevitable power, often
invoked against empirical evidence (as in specious debates on pedophilia and pornography). We must no longer refuse the sedition of
ordinary human bodies-in-sex.

Were we to follow this path, we might find that a new sexuality
exists not only in gay mens' lives but in others'. We may see, elsewhere, sexuality in modes of sociality that confound conventional
structural categories. We may begin to take seriously the sex experiences and activities of other peoples, places, and times. We may even
cease that pastoral project of which Bersani (1988) accuses us, stop
seeking to clean up sexuality in some liberal pluralist project of purification, and instead begin to enjoy a little more of the creative
potential in its sweat, bump, and grind.

References

Bersani, L. (1988). "Is the Rectum a Grave?" In Crimp, D. (ed.), *AIDS:
Cultural Analysis/Cultural Activism*. Cambridge, MA: MIT Press.
———. (1995). "Foucault, Freud, Fantasy, and Power." *GLQ*, 2(1/2):11–
33.
Bristow, J. (1989). "Homophobia/Misogyny: Sexual Fears, Sexual Defini-
tions." In Shepherd, S., and Wallis, M., (eds.), *Coming On Strong: Gay
Politics and Culture*. London: Unwin Hyman.
Coe, C. (1993). *Such Times*. Harmondsworth: Penguin Books.
Conigrave, T. (1995). *Holding the Man*. Ringwood Vic: McPhee Gribble
(Penguin Books).
Connell, R. W., and Dowsett, G. W. (1993). "The Unclean Motion of the
Generative Parts." In Connell, R. W., and Dowsett, G. W., (eds.), *Rethink-
ing Sex: Social Theory and Sexuality Research*. Philadelphia: Temple Uni-
versity Press.
Dowsett, G. W. (1996). *Practicing Desire: Homosexual Sex in the Era of
AIDS*. Stanford: Stanford University Press.

Maffesoli, M. (1991). "The Ethics of Aesthetics." *Theory, Culture & Society*, 8(1):7–20.

Moore, O. (1991). *A Matter of Life and Sex*. Harmondsworth: Penguin Books.

Rechy, J. (1977). *The Sexual Outlaw: A Documentary*. New York: Grove Weidenfeld.

Sedgwick, E. K. (1990). *Epistemology of the Closet*. Berkeley and Los Angeles: University of California Press.

Watney, S. (1986). "The Banality of Gender." *Oxford Literary Review*, 8(1/2):13–21.

Weeks, J. (1985). *Sexuality and Its Discontents: Meanings, Myths and Modern Sexualities*. London: Routledge and Kegan Paul.

Chapter Two

Masculinity in Indonesia

Genders, Sexualities, and Identities in a Changing Society

Dédé Oetomo

There is currently increasing use of the term and concept "gender" among Indonesian academics, primarily though not exclusively among those attached to centers for women's studies (established in major state universities as projects of the Office of the State Minister for Women's Affairs), and among activists for non-government organizations (NGOs) and community-based organizations (CBOs) working in the area of reproductive health. Much of this work on gender has focused disproportionately on women, with men figuring only, if at all, as the "equal and harmonious partners of women" (implicitly, but often also explicitly, limited to the realm of heterosexual marriage and family). At the same time, the term "gender" is often used as a synonym for "women" or euphemism for "feminism" or "feminist," with men not even discussed. While most of these academics and activists are concerned with how femininity is constructed, rarely if ever is the construction of masculinity discussed, let alone questioned.[1] Therefore, while femininity is a marked category, masculinity is unmarked. Another problem in Indonesian gender studies is its disregard for the *banci* and *waria*, who belong to what I have elsewhere termed a third gender (Oetomo, 1991b, 1996).[2] Together with the almost total silence around homosexualities, the omission of discussions around masculinity and the *banci* or *waria* gender identity and sexuality are blind spots in current gender studies in Indonesia.

I shall attempt to throw light on these blind spots by analyzing masculinity in a more nuanced manner, looking into diverse manifestations in different segments of Indonesian society. More specifically, I shall do this through a discussion of male sexualities in which I concretely demonstrate the construction of masculinity vis-à-vis not

46

only women but also waria and other men, whether or not homosexually identified.

I have gained my insights into issues of genders, sexualities, and identities in Indonesia through participant observation in waria and gay communities in Surabaya, where I have resided and worked since 1981. In addition, through working in gay activism during this same time, and in HIV/AIDS prevention since 1989, I have been able to carry out periodic observations in many other localities in Indonesia, broadening the range of sexualities observed.

Indonesian society is complex and diverse, composed of many social groups, all influenced in one way or another by capitalist development in its various guises since colonial times. The Indonesian middle class has been particularly influenced by this colonial history, with the resultant development of a middle-class sexual morality that resembles Victorian morality (see Onghokham, 1991). This morality figures strongly in the disregard, mentioned above, of the issues of waria and homosexual genders, sexualities, and identities. One must hasten to qualify, though, that under this veneer of prudery one still easily finds the pre-colonial richness of gender constructions, sexualities, and identities, especially among people from the working class. In this brief essay, I shall be able only to touch, in my illustrations,[3] on some of that richness.

In the remainder of this chapter, I shall delve into the complexities of masculine gender constructions by (1) looking at general public perceptions of "banci/waria"[4] gender identities and sexualities as an alternative way of looking at masculinity, and (2) examining the gender/sexual construction of banci/waria and gay-identified men. In so doing, I hope to throw more light onto masculine gender constructions in Indonesia.

"Banci/Waria" as Perceived by the General Public in Indonesia

Any member of Indonesian society is familiar with people referred to as "banci" or "waria,"[5] and these words are part of any Indonesian's vocabulary. Who are these "banci," in the perception of the general public, and when is this label applied?

To begin, someone is labeled "banci" when s/he appears androgynous in dress, physical features, or both, or behaves androgynously.

Very young children already identify certain appearances and behaviors as "banci," and parents often use the word to label their children who cross gender boundaries. Thus, when a boy plays with dolls or a girl climbs trees, s/he may be admonished by being called "banci" or told s/he is "banci" or "banci"-like (in the case of gender-noncomforming girls, the word *tomboy* is increasingly used as well, but with less negative connotation). The general public also identifies as "banci/waria" someone who hangs out on the streets and/or engages in sex. Some Indonesians further label many male fashion models and some male popular singers, along with female taxi drivers, bus conductors, athletes, policewomen, and the like, as at least "banci"-like.

Non-gender-conforming homosexually identified males are also identified as "banci/waria" by knowing neighbors and workmates. For many Indonesians, the category "homosexual" or "gay" is just not known, although one must hasten to add that, due to the increasing intensity of discourses around HIV/AIDS and homosexuality in the media, the words "homo," "homoseks," "homoseksual," "homoseksualitas," and "gay" have increasingly become known to those with media access. Nevertheless, it is my impression that, even among these persons, few know any real-life homo or gay persons, and hence most have at best a vague idea of whom the terms refer to. This situation is certainly quite different from general acquaintance and knowledge regarding "waria" (a term which, as mentioned earlier, may well include men who identify themselves as "homo" or "gay").

The stereotype that many Indonesians have about "waria" is that they are sexually impotent and/or have subnormally small or shriveled genitals. While it is true that a very small number of waria are pseudo-hermaphrodites, the stereotype does not hold water; a man who has sex with a waria is sometimes embarrassed to find that his penis is considerably smaller than that of his waria partner.

The category "banci/waria" does not, for the general public, necessarily connote sexual orientation. It is rather a label for nonconforming gender behavior or for a gender identity. In fact, except the streetwise, average Indonesians are ignorant of waria sexual behavior. That a secondary meaning of the word "banci" is "impotent" indicates that, in the mind of many Indonesians, banci are asexual beings. To these Indonesians, the mere information that "banci/waria" are engaged in sexual behavior is usually taken with great surprise. Also, the epithet "banci" is used to derogate men seen as "wishy-washy" and cowardly. Student or mass organizations considered not courageous enough to take part in actions critical of the government, for example, are often sent parcels containing bras, panties, lipstick, and a powder case.

As much as the general Indonesian public derogates "banci/waria," it also tolerates them to a considerable extent. Children and young men may bother a "waria" passing through their neighborhood, but never one who lives and is known in their own community. Young men sometimes touch or pinch a passing "waria" on different parts of the body and make sexual passes at her. At societal functions, "waria" are often asked to entertain; even parties held by the armed forces have been known to feature "waria" troupes, sometimes to the exclusion of other entertainers. Women like to have their hair done or faces made up in salons by "waria." In some neighborhoods, "waria" give cooking, sewing, embroidery, or hairdressing lessons to women in PKK meetings[6] or teach women about modern etiquette and personality development.

Sex with waria is certainly part of the sexual repertoire of Indonesian men, especially among the urban working class. These men know how to respond to a waria, even when the latter shows such masculine characteristics as a moustache or short hair (this applies as well to encounters with a homosexually identified man, or a man in transition to becoming a full-fledged waria). Only a few very naive men do not know that waria are genitally male (since most waria prefer not to have a sex-change operation) and once in bed are turned off to find that they are having sex with "a man dressed as a woman." Most men who actually have sex with waria fully know it is not a woman they are sleeping with; some even form lasting relationships with waria.

At this point, it may be relevant to ask how the men who have sex or form romantic relationships with waria perceive their own sexuality. I propose that, for them, it is rather *sexualities*. Their sexualities are diverse and fluid, and we must make a distinction between sexuality with women and sexuality with waria (and perhaps even men).

For Muslim men, for instance, sex with women outside marriage is considered *zinah* (adulterous), but this is not necessarily true of sex with waria. At least waria are, as it were, outside the realm of the serious sexuality proscribed except within marriage. Often, sex with waria is even perceived as "safer" and "cleaner," since it does not result in pregnancy, which carries certain socioeconomic responsibilities, and is perceived not to transmit commonly known STDs such as syphilis and gonorrhea.

It is important to note that in sexual intercourse, often the waria is the penetrator in anal and oral sex—and not only because the waria is aggressively seeking penetrative sex (see Oetomo, 1991b). Still, some waria can be aggressive in pursuing their men—a practice normally considered unfeminine in women—grabbing men by their arms, shoulders, hips, or even crotch. It is cases like these that make one think not all waria are consistently so-called "imitators of women." Their gender identity is, as it were, situational; waria vary between socially and culturally stereotyped masculine and feminine behavior according to whom they are with, need to avoid danger (such as police raids), and sorts of events they are involved in. Waria comedians, for instance, always make their audience laugh by slipping into masculine behavior while looking feminine.

The power dynamics of sexual and romantic relations between waria and men are complex and depend on many factors. In sexual intercourse, the penetrator waria more often than not plays the dominant role. This could result from a waria's larger physique or greater strength, or if the waria is older than her male sexual partners. It could also be based on a waria's stronger financial power; higher-income waria may penetrate poorer men because the waria are paying for the sexual favor or because the poorer men cannot pay for the encounter and hence must submit to the wishes of the waria. In romantic relations, too, often age and financial considerations come into play. Younger or poorer men can be "kept" by older or wealthier waria.

What is interesting is that the waria-loving men do not identify themselves as, and refuse to be termed, homosexual. They actually form an unmarked, nameless category. If they know of "homosexuals" ("homo") at all, they perceive these latter as men who have sex with males usually more Westernized, more middle class, wealthier, more likely to hang out at expensive discos, and so on. I therefore suggest that we are dealing with a difference in social construction between two socioeconomic groups in Indonesian society; the "waria" is a working-class construction and the "homo" a middle-class construction. In a similar way, we can see the former as a traditional construction and the latter as a modern construction.

Let us now consider how "waria" are perceived by Muslim Indonesians of the *santri* type.[7] While they know as much of the existence of "waria," and share the same construction of them as the rest of society, santri tend to approve of them less, referring to the Qur'ānic concept *khuntsa*, an in-between gendered person whose behavior is condemned. Among orthodox Nahdlatul Ulama Muslims in rural Java, homosexual relations (known as *amrot-amrotan*, "to play woman") between male pupils and *musyahaqah* ("female same-sex relations") between female pupils of *pesantren* (boarding schools) are condoned and tolerated, even institutionalized, as part of the learning process, and homosexual relations between adults are quietly accepted. (For a fuller account, see Oetomo, 1991a.) The younger partner in an *amrot-amortan*, often called the *amrot* ("woman") or *mairil* ("younger study-mate, friend, lover"), is usually an androgynous-looking younger boy. The adjective *muhanits* ("cute, androgynous, puerile") is used to describe the facial appearance of such boys, with the prominent distinguishing factor a downy, first-growth moustache. Very non-gender-conforming boys, who in the *abangan* world will be considered a "waria," have a very hard time in the *pesantren* context because they are teased and bothered by the other boys. It must be mentioned, though, that it is known that one does come across santri youths seducing "waria," whether for play or in seriousness; also, in waria communities, there are members with devout Islamic backgrounds.

Finally, it is pertinent to touch upon how the Indonesian state perceives "waria" and how it acts upon that perception. Officially, the dominant gender ideology of the Indonesian state recognizes only two genders, masculine and feminine, and in explicit expositions about these two genders, recognizes the principle of gender equality—albeit with fixed roles prescribed for men and women (as mentioned at the beginning of this paper). There is no mention of the existence, let alone the possibility, of a third gender such as the waria. The reality, however, is more complex. Since the beginning of the Suharto regime's rule, in the second half of the 1960s,[8] local governments—usually through the departments of social welfare—have given recognition to waria in the forms of subsidies for their activities, typically centering around hairdressing, sewing, and embroidery;[9] of approving the formation of associations and funding association activities; and of inclusion in certain festivities. More recently, a subordinate organization of the government party Musyawarah Kekeluargaan Gotong

Royong (MKGR), chaired by the State Minister for Women's Affairs, Mme. Mien Sugandhi, encouraged the formation of waria associations at the national, provincial, and district levels. In more than one locality, the sometimes baffled MKGR has also attempted to recruit gay-identified men. My guess is that the organized waria will be used in political campaigns, since many are entertainers and all are popular in large gatherings composed primarily of men. In the political campaigning prior to the 1992 general elections, the rival Indonesian Democratic Party (PDI) was supported by a few gay entertainers and artists, at least some of whom were known as gay by the young men and women who adored their live and TV performances. At that time, PDI gained a considerable vote attributed to young people.

As for lesbians and gay men, the state ideology again contains no explicit mention of them. In practice, while individual closeted male homosexuals can go very far in government careers, in the framework of HIV/AIDS work, at least at the national level, the small Indonesian gay network has been consistently excluded from government-sponsored committees since 1993. It is clear that organized, *out*, gay men are disapproved of by the government. The State Minister for Population, Professor Haryono Suyono, chair of the National Family Planning Coordinating Board, made statements disapproving of homosexuality and, more specifically, of same-sex marriages, on several occasions, notably in the context of the International Conference for Population and Development in Cairo in September 1994. He has also spoken adamantly against the concept of sexual health for Indonesian society. Another government official, the previously mentioned Mme. Sugandhi, issued a statement disapproving of lesbians, on the occasion of the Asia/Pacific preparatory meeting for the 1995 Beijing International Conference on Women. Although she recognized that in the West lesbians exist and are demanding their rights, and that lesbians might have a place in an international conference, she precluded such a possibility for Indonesia. One wonders if and how much these two officials know about the definite homosexuality of at least one colleague in the cabinet, or about the rumored homosexuality of others. My guess is that, in such a totalitarian regime, the powers-that-be surely know such intimate details—but apparently these do not matter. To sum up, the perception of the state concerning waria identity and sexuality is, I believe, in accordance with that of the general public.

Waria and Gay-Identified Men in Their Own Perception

Within waria and gay communities themselves, there prevails a construction different from that of the general public and the state. There is, first, an almost watertight distinction between the categories "banci/waria" and "gay," at least superficially and in most cases. This categorical separation is mirrored at the level of social interaction. In some places, there is hardly any contact between waria and gay communities, which form separate communities with different hangouts. In some localities, there may even be hostility between the two communities at the street level. Waria, many of whom sell sexual services to men, may accuse gay men of paying the same men for sex, thus taking away business. There seems to be a correlation between socioeconomic status and identification as waria or gay. Waria are mostly working class or from working-class families, while most gay men either hail from middle-class families or aspire to climb to the middle class.

If we look more closely, however, we find borderline cases—gay men who assume a waria identity (or, at least, appearance) in certain contexts, and the reverse. A gay man might cross-dress at night, for example, or when cruising in another town or hangout. A person who assumes a waria appearance or identity only at night does so from professional constraints (for example, the dress code at a place of work may not allow males to wear female clothing) or if not entirely sure of wanting to become waria totally. Gay men who cross-dress in another town or hangout do so, however, for tactical reasons; they believe that by looking like a waria it is easier to lure men into having sex, especially since, as we saw earlier, the society at large is not familiar with the "gay" category.

In fact, it is safe to say that becoming a total waria is usually a process. Adolescents who feel that they are "women trapped in men's bodies" often start cross-dressing only occasionally, for parties and similar events, and gradually do so more often, until finally they cross-dress all the time. Becoming a waria is similar to the gay coming-out process; there are often conflicts with parents and relatives, some never resolved. The reverse process—that of banci gradually assuming a gay male identity—is also possible, though much less common.

The Construction of Gender among Waria and Gay Men

Waria

Waria perceive themselves as a third gender, in addition to *laki* or *laki-laki* ("male") and *perempuan* ("female"). As mentioned earlier, many describe themselves as "women trapped in men's bodies" and see themselves as embodying elements of both maleness and femaleness. In fact, there is a range of waria gender behavioral characteristics, from the waria who acts and adopts the refined, coy (*halus*) characteristics of the "proper" woman to the banci who adopts the coarse, outgoing (*kasar*) characteristics of the typical lower-class man. The contrast between feminine dress and masculine behavior in some banci can be quite remarkable. This is especially so in middle-age waria, who may adopt the image of the *ibu-biu* ("matron") but at times show very *kasar* behavior; they raise their leg to show their panties, scratch their crotches, pretend to fellate microphones, or punch young men very hard. Waria of the *kasar* type generally serve as protectors of their *halus* friends, and may beat up younger, physically weaker men for not paying enough for sexual services or for pestering the weaker friends.

It is interesting that some leaders of the grassroots waria movement, notably Panky Kenthut of the Surabaya Association of Waria, have repeatedly demanded recognition of a third gender—so far without any clear response from the authorities, although some waria have been able to have the gender entry *laki-laki* (waria) written on their identity cards (at the most, a discretionary policy at the local, ward level). At Surbaya's Taman Remaja, an amusement park where there are waria musical shows every Thursday night, the public toilets are designated *"wanita"* ("ladies") and *"pria/waria"* ("gentlemen/waria"). Among other unsettled issues is the question of what to wear when praying as Muslims; some waria believe they are basically men and hence discard "female" appearance before God, while others (including, obviously, those who have undergone a sex-change operation) go all the way and wear the *mukena* (prayer shroud) required of women. Another issue is whether or not to have a sex-change operation. While for most waria this comes down primarily to a question of prohibitive cost (the least expensive operation can cost Rps6 million [approximately U.S.$3,000 at the time of writing], not counting the counseling and the series of silicone and hormonal injections prior to surgery), some who could afford the operation nonetheless disapprove of it, arguing that through a sex-change operation one becomes only superficially a woman. Many who prefer not to have a sex-change operation also state that they still cherish their penis, which they like to use to penetrate men.

Professionally, waria typically engage in feminine activities such as hairdressing and makeup, embroidery, and cooking. But they also carry out gender-neutral activities, becoming a shaman, for instance, or a comedian (without cashing in on waria identity). In this regard, too, the most appropriate way to characterize the construction of the waria identity in Indonesian society would be as a third gender that incorporates both maleness and femaleness. This, I believe, is further corroborated by the way waria perceive men and women.

Gay men, whom we shall discuss in a moment, often jokingly call themselves *perempuan* ("female") or ask each other how advanced their "pregnancy" is, but waria very rarely do. In fact, many who have had a sex-change operation still consider themselves waria and hang out with non-operated friends. At least in Java, they also call women *racun* ("poison"), having seen their men leave them for women. A very few waria, however, are married and have children, and some others have sexual or romantic relations with lesbians. Finally, a very few waria have sex with one another, although, generally speaking, this is considered aberrant.

Waria divide men into two categories: the *laki* ("men"), or *laki asli* ("real men"), and the gay men. The great majority are not interested in having sex or forming relationships with men they perceive as gay. But two significant phenomena must be highlighted: the more *kasar* banci often aggressively pursue their men, and once they decide to have sex, the laki asli may willingly and even eagerly ask to be the penetratee (anally and orally).

To conclude this section on waria gender construction, it must be emphasized that the category is not one in which sexual orientation is prominent, unless of course one modifies the homosexual-heterosexual range by adding waria-oriented sexuality to it.

Gay Men

The construction of gender among some gay men is similar to that among waria. They have the same construct "laki asli," which refers to men who act masculinely and whom they do not consider gay. The difference from the waria construction lies in the fact that gay men regard themselves as men (albeit not so "genuine"). Stereotypically, the laki asli are the penetrators in sex and usually refuse to do wet kissing.[10] Indeed, some just lie down and do nothing, usually when being fellated but also during anal sex (i.e., with the gay-identified partner sitting on the man's penis)—an interesting fact, since the general public considers it women who are supposed to remain passive. Obviously, there are variations; the laki asli who acts masculinely in public may willingly and eagerly be the penetratee in sex. Many gay men accept this behavior, but a small number immediately lose interest as soon as they find their laki asli are as "gay" as themselves. The presence of sustained erection in a lakli asli when having sex with a gay man is not considered a marker of gayness. Some laki asli are trade, basically heterosexual men who perform sex with gay men for the money. In fact, some gay men refuse to have sex with men who are not trade and/or prefer men who are heterosexually married.

I would hypothesize that gay men who have sex only with laki asli tend to be nearer the low end of the middle class. Other gay men, who tend to be more educated and better off economically, prefer fellow gay men, even those who are non-gender-conforming. Those who disapprove of gay men having sex with one another call such sex "lesbian sex" (*lesbongan*), sex between two "women."[11] In contrast, the past decade has seen a trend in larger cities of gay men attending exercise gyms and priding themselves on their muscular development; these middle-class men tend to prefer each other for sexual relationships and to loathe feminine behavior.

Many gay men have two constructions of femaleness, the *perempuan* (or *wanita*) and the *racun*. Gay men tend to look at "real women" as *racun* for the same reason that waria do. The word also refers to "wife." This seems to signify a rather strong misogyny.

Married gay men, however, do not generally refer to their wives as *racun*. At the same time, their discourse is full of expressions that jokingly refer to themselves as "women." They talk about becoming pregnant or about being abandoned or loved by their husbands, and desire to purchase artificial female genitals or hairbuns. In some long-term relationships between gay-identified men and laki asli, the laki asli husbands, far from being the typical husband who provides economically, are financially dependent on the gay-identified men.

Conclusion

The above discussion of constructions of waria and gay-identified men, among both the general public and waria and gay men themselves, reveals what I believe is a richer, more nuanced picture of masculinity in Indonesia than is present in most academic and activist accounts. It should be clear now that not only must one seriously consider *men* in Indonesian gender studies (i.e., not exclusively focus on women), one must also consider "men" as constructed in a complex manner. For example, in some (generally public) contexts, especially in relations with women, men can, indeed, be dominant, but in other, more private contexts, and in relations with waria or gay-identified men, issues of class distinction, age difference, and, in general, unequal power relations must be taken into consideration to understand domination. Domination, that is, is not necessarily and absolutely a function of gender differences, but is perhaps as greatly a function of class distinctions, age differences, and unequal power generally.

Notes

1. One can make inadequate inferences, at best, about Indonesian masculinity from the criticisms voiced of inequalities between women and men. The portrait that emerges is of men always acting as heads of families and as breadwinners, operating in the public sphere, and not being responsible for the upbringing of children or the sharing of household work. In the area of sexuality, one would infer a thinly disguised "legendary" heterosexual promiscuity of men and a consistent role of men as initiators and dominators in heterosexual intercourse.

2. "Banci" is the original Indonesia word referring to people of the third gender and their characteristics. "Waria" is a euphemistic, emancipatory ab-

breviation coined in the late 1970s from the polite Indonesian words for "woman" and for "man," *pria*. Earlier, in the 1960s, a similar abbreviation, *wadam*, was coined from *wanita* and *Adam*; criticized by some Islamic leaders in the 1970s, this was replaced by the new abbreviation. Throughout this paper I shall generally use "waria" since this is the term preferred by the subjects themselves in formal discourse, but where necessary, I shall use "banci."

3. For a fairly extensive survey of homosexually related diversity in genders and sexualities in Indonesia, see Oetomo, 1991a.

4. A notational convention: Whenever I refer to the category *banci* or *waria* as perceived by the general public (i.e., people who are not themselves *waria* or gay identified), I shall write the word between quotation marks, thus: *"banci"* or *"waria."* Otherwise, I am referring to the category as perceived by *waria* themselves and by gay-identified men.

5. Alternatively, Indonesians refer to these people by the slang word *bencong*, or by the various words known in different regional vernaculars, such as *wandu* (Javanese), *bandhu* (Madurese), and *kawe-kawe* (Buginese).

6. PKK stands for Pendidikan Kesejahteraan Keluarga (Family Welfare Education). It is a government-encouraged neighborhood wives' organization set up in all neighborhoods in Indonesia, with programs emphasizing the femininity of wives and mothers (Suryakusuma, 1991).

7. The *santri-abangan* religious dichotomy, which Clifford Geertz introduced based on his study of Javanese society (Geertz, 1960), while perhaps not so clearcut anymore, can, in my opinion, still be used to make a distinction between the traditionally less syncretic Muslims (*santri*) and the more syncretic (*abangan*).

8. The militaristic New Order regime came into power in 1966 in the aftermath of an abortive coup allegedly masterminded by the Indonesian Communist Party on 1 October 1965. The first few years of its rule were characterized by a loosening of what was previously restricted or banned, such as Westernized, international popular culture.

9. The same skills, often with the addition of religious lessons, are also given to female sex trade workers in so-called rehabilitation centers run by the Department of Social Welfare. The idea is that these skills will equip women for earning income as respectable citizens.

10. This is due partly to the view, especially among some working-class people, that deep kissing is disgusting and only practiced by Westerners, and partly to the belief among some working-class men that deep kissing is only for one's girlfriend. The class distinction is significant: most of the laki asli hail from the working class.

11. Other terms in Indonesian gay slang for such behavior are *bathokan* or *tari tempurung* ("to play [dance] with coconut shells [women's breasts]"), *tari-tarian* ("to dance with each other"—referring to the two gay partners'

feminine behavior), and *kartinian* ("to play Kartini"—Kartini being an early women's emancipation figure).

References

Geertz, C. (1960). *The Religion of Java*. Glencoe, IL: The Free Press.

Oetomo, D. (1991a). "Homoseksualitas di Indonesia." *Prisma*, 20, no. 7 (July), 84–96.

———. (1991b). "Patterns of Bisexuality in Indonesia." In Tielman, R. A. P., Carballo, M., and Hendriks, A. C. (eds.), *Bisexuality and HIV/AIDS: A Global Perspective*, 119–126. Buffalo, NY: Prometheus.

———. (1996). "Gender and Sexual Orientation in Indonesia." In Laurie Jo Sears (ed.), *Fantasizing the Feminine in Indonesia*. Durham, NC: Duke University Press.

Onghokham. 1991. "Kekuasaan dan Seksualitas: Lintasan Sejarah Pra dan Masa Kolonial." *Prisma*, 20, no. 7 (July), 15–23.

Suryakusuma, J. I. (1991). "Seksualitas dalam Pengaturan Negara." *Prisma*, 20, no. 7 (July), 70–83.

Chapter Three

Male Homosexuality
and Seropositivity

The Construction of Social Identities in Brazil

Veriano Terto Jr.

In the following pages, I will discuss a number of issues concerning the impact of AIDS on Brazilian male homosexuals. This impact is not limited to the consequences of AIDS as a medical phenomenon, but is a broad sociocultural phenomenon affecting the lives of millions of people individually and collectively.

The link between AIDS and homosexuality dates to the first years of the epidemic, when U.S. scientists, perceiving the epidemic as a problem of homosexual men, gave it the name "Gay Related Immunodeficiency" (GRID). AIDS arrived in Brazil in 1981, when sensational newspaper headlines announced the arrival of a "gay plague" even though there were no officially reported cases in Brazil that year (Daniel and Míccolis, 1983; Daniel and Parker, 1991, 1993). Only in 1982 were the first cases of AIDS officially registered.

As in many other countries during the same period, old prejudices against homosexuality were reinforced and extreme and violent actions taken against homosexuals, since the latter were considered responsible for the illness. Today, more than fifteen years after the advent of AIDS as an epidemic in the West, the voices of those who blame homosexual individuals for spreading AIDS to other population strata remain strong.

In most Latin American countries, homosexual transmission remains responsible for up to fifty percent of AIDS cases. In Brazil, the percentage of cases linked to homosexual transmission has been stabilizing in recent years, especially in regard to new infections (Harrad, 1995; Parker, 1994). However, this does not mean that the association between AIDS and male homosexuality should receive less attention, since the majority of AIDS patients in hospitals still is comprised of male homosexuals, and many people continue to consider AIDS a punishment for homosexual practices—anal sex, in particular.

This recent stabilization of the number of new AIDS cases registered in official epidemiological statistics contrasts with the difficulties and prejudices faced in daily life by men who have sex with men. Moreover, AIDS prevention projects aimed at this population are still relatively rare in Brazil, and few health service providers are ready to discuss and face the homophobia that effectively denies these men adequate medical care. Despite the gravity of the AIDS epidemic among the male homosexual population, no Latin American government has responded effectively to this problem, either through creation of prevention programs or through recognition of the contributions made by homosexual groups and individuals through community mobilization, education, activism, and care for those already ill.

The association between AIDS and homosexuality raises serious problems, from the personal to the judicial. With the advance of the epidemic, many homosexual couples have been hit by a discriminatory legal system that does not recognize their relationships and hinders partners from leaving inheritances to their companions or sharing health insurance, and from other rights enjoyed by heterosexual couples. The issue of violence against homosexuals—worsened by prejudices—also needs society's attention, since the impunity granted these actions reinforces the vulnerability and marginalization of homosexuals and the continued violation of their citizenship. During the last few years, Brazilian gay groups have been documenting cases of such violence and denouncing both the impunity of the aggressors and the negligence of Brazilian authorities toward investigating these crimes (Mott, 1997). For example, *travestis* (transvestites) have became easy targets for attack by homophobic gangs on the outskirts of many large cities—with the justification almost always that the travestis are spreading AIDS to the general population and thus should be eliminated. The increase in these attacks, as well as the vulnerability of *travestis* to HIV, recently led to formation of the first organizations of travestis who seek, besides AIDS prevention, to denounce this violence and to advocate for their own civil rights. These organizations include the *Esperança* (Hope) Group in Curitiba, the *TULIPA* (or TULIP, an acronym that in Portuguese means United Transvestites and Transformers Fighting Relentlessly for the Prevention of

AIDS) Group in Santo André, São Paulo, and *ASTRAL* (Association of Transvestites and Liberated Persons) in Rio de Janeiro.

But before going on to discuss the ways AIDS has transformed the experiences and identities of homosexual and bisexual men in Brazil, it is worth taking a few steps back to briefly describe the context in which the epidemic arrived—the many rapid and important changes taking place in Brazilian life, and in the social organization of homosexuality in Brazil, during the late 1970s and early 1980s.

Brazilian Homosexualities Before the Time of AIDS

AIDS arrived in Brazil during a decade when the country was emerging from a twenty-year military dictatorship and Brazilian society was searching for new paths within the parameters of the modern democracies in the West. Within a wider political opening during the early 1980s, the first Brazilian gay groups emerged in the major cities and fought for the right to be different and for the affirmation of homosexual identities. These local groups, although quite diverse in terms of political philosophy and practice, reached out to one another, culminating in the First Brazilian Meeting of Homosexuals in São Paulo in 1979, which brought together representatives from many regions of Brazil; a second national meeting was held the following year in Rio de Janeiro. The emerging Homosexual Movement (*Movimento Homossexual*) grew parallel to, and attempted to form alliances with, other minority organizations and movements of the period (the women's movement, Afro-Brazilian movement, and ecology movement, among others) that shared a concern with democracy, acceptance, and social justice (see MacRae, 1990). For example, the São Paulo *Somos* Group (literally, "We Are"), an important gay group of the time, participated in the 1982 public manifestations against the Argentine dictatorship, one of the most repressive and homophobic Latin American regimes of the 1970s and 1980s; other homosexual groups participated with São Paulo industrial workers' unions in First of May, or International Workers' Day, commemorations (Trevisan, 1986). The Homosexual Movement also took part in discussions at the National Congress for the defense of changes in the constitution that would benefit or even guarantee homosexuals' rights (da Silva, 1993). These actions illustrate the sociopolitical changes in Brazil around this time—and they also ultimately contributed to a greater visibility for homosexuals and to the construction of other social representations of homosexuals—not only as political actors claiming citizenship but also as potential consumers in an emerging consumer market (Parker, 1999).

In the larger Brazilian cities, there was a rapid proliferation of commercial gay meeting places, such as bars, saunas, and discos, superimposed over the more clandestine, or underground, circuits of movie theaters, parks, streets, and other "spots" for homosexual encounters. Homosexuals not only became more visible as they conquered new spaces, they achieved greater social and economic status as "demanding" consumers with "good purchasing power" who deserved networks of specialized services such as travel agencies, hotels, clinics, and so on. There were no longer only "crazy queers," exotic and obligatory characters in samba "schools" (groups organized for Carnival parades), or travestis who appeared in places of prostitution and the crime reports of the sensational press; rather, new and elaborated cultural representations of male homosexuality appeared—through an interplay of activists, political groups, books, academic theses, favorable municipal laws, and artistic expression, all shedding light on life styles and possibilities of "being homosexual" far from the realms of the exotic, the forbidden, the "ill." Such changes were decisive for the next generation of male homosexuals, who, in spite of the advent of AIDS and related intensification of prejudice, continued to participate in the growing gay (sub)culture and to create new representations of homosexuality in Brazilian society (Parker, 1999).

These new times and new visibility can be seen by the end of the 1970s and beginning of the 1980s in the gay newspaper *Lampião* (*Torch*), distributed at newsstands, which served as a vehicle for expressing the main ideas, as well as the impasses, of the Homosexual Movement. During this same period, the important ex-guerrilla fighters and activists Fernando Gabeira and Herbert Daniel returned from exile and brought issues of (homo)sexuality into public discourse in Brazil in an unprecedented way—indeed, Daniel was the last political exile of the dictatorship to return to the country and, in the Brazilian left, his literary works and political essays raised heated discussions of sexuality and homosexuality (Daniel and Míccolis, 1983). At much the same time, Argentine poet and anthropologist Nestor Perlongher, escaping from the homophobic fury of his country's dictatorship, arrived at the University of Campinas and, with fellow anthropologists Edward MacRae and Peter Fry, brought a new dimension to academic research on homosexuality in Brazil (see for example Fry, 1982; Fry and MacRae, 1983; Perlongher, 1987a, 1987b). In more popular culture, the era was marked by the media success of travesti Roberta Close, who became a national sex symbol in the early 1980s (Parker, 1999; Perlongher, 1987b). One decade later, Daniel would die from AIDS-related complications, but not before leaving a decisive contribution to the organization of community response to the challenge posed by the epidemic. AIDS would also take countless other key figures working on homosexuality in the Brazilian context, among them Perlongher (in 1992).

To understand the changes in Brazilian homosexualities, it is important to note that men who have sex with men in Brazil have never lacked—in regard to sex—places for encounters in the larger cities; among others, movie-theaters, public bathrooms, and parks long offered a haven for homoerotic activities. The liberalism of the late 1970s produced new places and different forms of encounters, in which sexual play was not necessarily the key note. Bars, activist organizations, and recreational gay groups offered possibilities of other ways of relating, new opportunities for overcoming an often oppressive clandestinity. As in many other countries (see for example Herdt and Boxer, 1991), gay groups in Brazil made a decisive contribution toward more positive attitudes on homosexuality and for political activism around the civil rights of "minorities."

During the 1980s, the number of clandestine locales decreased in cities such as Rio de Janeiro and São Paulo. AIDS and the resultant new wave of prejudice should not, however, be considered the only factors responsible for this change; there were also: reinforcement of the commercial gay network, including more institutionalized meeting places; more police repression in the streets; changes in urban spaces, resulting from reforms and more lighting of parks, streets, and gardens; the growing violence of armed robberies; and the economic crisis, which increased poverty and the number of homeless people living in the streets. These factors contributed to the dismantling of most of the circuit of more orgiastic, anonymous, and clandestine sex typical of the (homo)sexual scenes of the 1970s (Terto, 1989).

Despite many commonalities with other countries in the ways

AIDS impacted homosexuality—among them, the symbolic association "AIDS = homosexuality," the wave of prejudices unleashed by
the epidemic, and the similar epidemiologic pattern—several factors
distinguish the Brazilian experience from that of the U.S. and Western
Europe. In Brazil, there was no gay subculture as organized and visible as those in the Northern Hemisphere or in Australia. And, as
mentioned earlier, AIDS arrived in the midst of a moment of intense
sociopolitical change and strong popular movements that facilitated
the denunciation of oppression and the organization of struggle for
civil rights and affirmation of difference among many marginalized
social sectors, including homosexuals. Nonetheless, it is important to
recognize that the changes in homosexuality in the large Brazilian
cities were strongly influenced by Northern Hemisphere homosexualities, through movies, music, tourism, fashion, international gay media, and the international (and, by extension, national) gay movement
(Parker, 1999). This influence also reinforced tendencies towards
other models of relationships as alternatives to the active–passive hi-
erarchical model typical of Latin American macho culture (Parker,
1991, 1999; Murray, 1992; Fry and MacRae, 1983). These new and
more egalitarian models broke with the culturally constituted assumption that a homosexual relationship would necessarily involve
one partner who penetrates—the "active" man, who enjoys a higher
social status—and one partner who is penetrated—the "passive" fairy,
who is socially despicable.

The influence of other ideologies, especially from the left, marked
the power of the progressive popular movements of the 1970s in Latin
America. By 1983, when AIDS began to be widely discussed in the
Brazilian media and in general society, the young Homosexual Movement (like other late-1970s identity movements) had suffered set-
backs, with most of its groups in process of extinction. As Brazil began
to emerge from its long period of authoritarian rule, political energy
and attention turned to broader national questions of redemocratization and direct democratic elections; more localized struggles
around issues such as gender, ethnicity, and sexuality were increasingly seen as secondary concerns within the political context of the
period (MacRae, 1990; Parker, 1999). Few gay groups formed in the
late 1970s or early 1980s survived to the 1990s. Despite this weakening of the movement, the homosexual group *"Outra Coisa"* ("Another Thing," or Something Else), with the public health authorities

of São Paulo, in July 1983 began distributing AIDS educational leaf-
lets and working on community prevention services. Such initiatives,
carried on in the following years by activists who had emerged from
the ranks of the Homosexual Movement, contributed decisively to
the creation of the *ONGs/AIDS* (AIDS/NGOs, nongovernmental organizations formed to work exclusively on AIDS), and to community
response to the HIV/AIDS epidemic. Among the most important of
these new organizations were, in the mid-1980s, GAPA/SP (Support
Group for Prevention of AIDS/São Paulo) founded in 1985, which
included many activists from the Homosexual Movement among its
leaders and membership, and ABIA (Brazilian Interdisciplinary AIDS
Association), founded in Rio de Janeiro in 1986, which included members of the gay group *Atobá* and other gay community representatives
and leaders. Indeed, from the mid-1980s on, the history of homosexuals in Brazil was marked by the irruption of the epidemic—and the
history of the epidemic, by the activism and involvement of homosexuals. In the following section, I will discuss some implications
raised by the HIV/AIDS epidemic for the homosexual or gay
(sub-)culture of the late 1980s.

Changing Homosexualities in Times
of AIDS

Considering the changes occurring in the last few years, and reviewing
the literature available on homosexuality in Brazil (Parker, 1991; Perlongher, 1987a; Fry and MacRae, 1983), one sees an enormous diversity of terms for men who have sex with men. Research conducted
in Brazil (Parker, Mota, and Lourenço, 1994; Parker and Terto, 1998)
shows that these multiple identities composing the mosaic of homosexual desires and lifestyles imply a greater or lesser degree of information about HIV and about forms of prevention, as well as different
ways of dealing with sexuality, otherness, and health. What is common
among those who identify themselves as gays, or men who have sex
with men, or queers, are only the erotic practices, prejudices, and
discrimination such desires provoke—including those related to
AIDS. This universe is much more diversified than the scientific concept of "homosexual," which, like the epidemiological concept "risk
group," seems to suggest a monolithic and homogeneous bloc, a single
population group. In fact, both in the social-science literature and in

daily life, we find homosexualities and pluralities linking sexuality to social class, ethnic group, economic status, serologic status, and other differences (Costa, 1992; Parker, 1999; Terto, 1997).

Presently, many researchers and educators involved with AIDS prevention and social research on male homosexuality increasingly seek to emphasize these pluralities in their planning, for several reasons: to confront concepts used by the medical-epidemiological field; to broaden the reach of their initiatives; to follow an international trend of pluralist nomenclature in educational and research projects. The plurality of homosexualities is observable in many countries (Altman, 1993), and this international perspective may be contributing to a broader vision of the relationship between AIDS and homosexualities.

The linking of AIDS with homosexuality has stirred intense debates worldwide. In the 1980s, many gay groups, including some in Brazil, tried not to get directly involved with the issue of AIDS, in order not to reinforce this association. At the same time, in Brazil as in other countries, emerging community responses to the epidemic were elicited by homosexual leaders or incipient gay organizations (Altman, 1993). Thus, AIDS came to strongly influence 1980s gay activism. On the one hand, there were groups who did not want to mix their struggles with the demands of the epidemic; most did not last long, whether for lack of resources or for failure to respond to the demands of a population increasingly hard-hit by the epidemic. They were also full of uncertainties to which their activism of differences and identities failed to respond. On the other hand, there were gay groups that incorporated AIDS as a problem to be faced and saw the possibility of reinforcing activism through the resources available for AIDS (Parker, 1999; Terto, 1997).

Most AIDS/NGOs created in Brazil in the 1980s were founded by homosexual men, and the main leadership of this movement comprised homosexual individuals. Despite the charismatic power of such members, and the transition of some from the gay movement to AIDS-related work, these organizations dedicated few efforts toward men who had sex with men, choosing instead to address a wider community (Altman, 1994). But even when de-emphasizing, or even avoiding, a direct position on the tragedy experienced by homosexuals (in some cases, by their own homosexual and seropositive leaders), these organizations opened a new field of activism, mobilized decisive community responses to the epidemic, and gave new dimensions to the visibility of homosexuality—no longer seen simply in terms of difference, or as an identity, but rather as referring to individuals equal to others, with the same rights and duties as other citizens (Carricaburu and Pierret, 1992).

Under the motto "AIDS is everybody's problem," used by many gay groups and AIDS/NGOs, activists tried to break the association "AIDS = homosexuality." The AIDS/NGOs did not want to be known as gay groups, an identity many AIDS activists felt could hinder their own more global engagement in the issue of AIDS and perhaps damage an organizations' image with the community at large and the funding agencies beginning to support AIDS-related work. Thus—in contrast to what happened in the early 1980s—in the late 1980s and early 1990s, homosexuality was banalized, no longer so important to claim or affirm. According to this new perspective, everybody, regardless of sexual preferences, lifestyles, habits, or the like, was equal when facing HIV, and deserved the same treatments, rights, and citizenship. The tension between this universalist perspective, which related the AIDS problem to other universal issues like human rights, versus the perspective focused on specificities—which considered priorities, vulnerabilities, identities, and needs—typified the agenda of most organizations and civil groups working with AIDS in Brazil. Even in the late 1990s, this tension between the "general" and the "particular" in the community's response to the epidemic is still observable in discussions of the concept "living with AIDS": does this concept apply to all who consider themselves vulnerable to the risk of HIV infection, or only to those seropositive to the virus? (see Terto, 1997).

Many homosexual individuals who had not identified with direct homosexual or gay activism found in the AIDS/NGOs an ideal space for social participation, in some cases motivated by philanthropy and altruism, for the definition of sexual identities was only one among other important concerns (Seffner, 1995; Terto, 1997). Other persons, previously distant from any social movement but strongly affected by the epidemic, started looking to the AIDS/NGOs for resources and social and psychological support to manage their daily lives. In many ways, the AIDS/NGOs became, together with the specifically gay groups, a reference for homosexual men (and perhaps, to a lesser extent, lesbians), especially for socialization and support.

The epidemic brought homosexuality into the open, forcing public administrations and medical institutions to acknowledge the existence of homosexual relationships, although recognition did not always result in concrete actions or benefits. Nonetheless, the visibility of homosexuality was amplified and occupied new spaces. In Brazil, as in other countries, gay groups were called upon to occupy seats in government committees for discussion and implementation of public policies for HIV/AIDS and STD prevention and care. International agencies, such as the World Health Organization (WHO), recommended that AIDS prevention should address homosexuals as well as other vulnerable populations, and homosexuality has not been considered a psychiatric disease since the 1980s. During national political campaigns and within political parties, candidates have emerged, particularly on the local level, who identify themselves as gay, support the claims of gay groups, and/or advocate for greater attention to the issue of AIDS by public administrations.

The effects of this visibility brought about by AIDS are open to debate, as little has been done concretely to minimize the consequences of the epidemic, and as violence, stigma, and discrimination against homosexuals continues, often supported by the media and popular opinion. In spite of the efforts of gay groups and AIDS/NGOs, insufficient public resources have gone to prevention and care for homosexuals. As suggested by Parker (1994), AIDS, although not essentially a homosexual problem, is nonetheless an issue especially important for homosexuals. This particularity needs to be considered. Under the pretext of "de-homosexualizing" the epidemic into "everybody's problem," many organizations, institutions, and sectors of society have ignored AIDS' effects on the male homosexual population. Although the epidemic does affect everybody in some way, and although everybody runs the risk of being infected by HIV, how AIDS affects homosexuals—as well as other social groups, such as hemophiliacs, injecting drug users, and sex workers—has its specificity. As shown by research carried out by Carricaburu and Pierret (1992) with male homosexuals, hemophiliacs, and heterosexuals, the history and social insertion of each group shaped the reactions and ways each perceived HIV and its consequences.

The vulnerability of homosexuals to HIV is intimately related to the stigma, discrimination, and marginality assigned to homosexuality. It is well known that individuals with low self-esteem, or fearing discrimination, or under the pressure of prejudices, do not seek help or adequate treatment—whether from fear, or from negligence toward self or others. Many people in Brazil still prefer to seek medical treatment for STDs in pharmacies and drugstores, rather than from health service providers, whose homophobic attitudes often submit a patient to stigma and embarrassment. Another concern is the thousands of men who, although living in heterosexual marriages, have extramarital relations with other men. The pressure of prejudices, aggravated by both a homosexuality and a family life not well defined, may reinforce HIV vulnerability of not only a man but a whole family.

Some AIDS/NGOs, such as ABIA, have tried to respond with intervention projects targeting men who have sex with men, and by establishing alliances with other AIDS organizations and gay groups. Most gay groups (for example, *Grupo Dignidade* [Dignity] in Curitiba or GGB [the *Grupo Gay de Bahia*] in Salvador) now see AIDS as a central question for their agenda; a meeting was organized during the seventh Brazilian Encounter of Homosexuals (Curitiba, January 1995) to discuss the impact of AIDS among homosexuals and homosexual participation in the struggle against the epidemic. In all of these initiatives a dilemma remains: how to develop AIDS prevention programs and activities for homosexuals, and to lessen the inroads of a tragedy affecting the lives of millions of men who have sex with men, yet not reinforce—on the contrary, to deconstruct—the stigmas associated with both homosexuality and AIDS. Ongoing dialogue between society at large and gay groups, AIDS/NGOs, public administrations, and institutions may result in the promotion of solidarity and the creation of positive sociocultural references about homosexuality, to the benefit of everyone.

In trying to deconstruct the "homosexuals' AIDS," with its representations of sin, deviation, promiscuity, and the like, so strongly marked since the beginning of the epidemic, it is important to respect not only the history of the tragedy, but also the effective responses of the gay community, including what is now called "safer sex," or the organization of self-help and activist groups, initially conceived by homosexual groups and individuals and greatly influencing many initiatives for prevention and care for *all* people. Around the world, gay groups have been among those at the forefront of responding to AIDS as a political phenomenon—not only an issue of public health to be resolved by technical solutions proposed by "experts" (Watney, 1993).

Living with the Epidemic

Ongoing research, initiated in 1989 by the Institute of Social Medicine at the State University of Rio de Janeiro together with ABIA, estimated that approximately 90 percent of those men having sex with men already knew about AIDS, about the ways HIV was transmitted, and about the means of preventing HIV infection (Parker, Mota, and Lourenço, 1994; Parker and Terto, 1998). What the findings of this research may also indicate—besides identification of risks and means of prevention—is how people live with the epidemic. This can be especially important information for the implementation of prevention projects, and for the definition of public health policies that can consider the realities of the homosexual population. What ideas about prevention should be explored with these men? What in fact are they being helped to prevent (since AIDS may already be a tragic reality in their daily lives)? Whether through having infected or ill friends or partners, or having been tested for HIV, or fear of being infected, or adoption of safer practices (with the doubts raised by such changes), or through the uncertainty shrouding the future, this population already has more in common than homoerotic desires or shared identities. It shares the experience of having to live with the epidemic (Terto, 1997).

French authors (for instance, Pollak, 1993; Carricaburu and Pierret, 1992) indicate that uncertainties regarding the recommendations about safer sex, the contradictions and lack of precision of scientific discourse, and the search for resources to address issues imposed by the epidemic, are proven factors in bringing together this population, perhaps more than are issues concerning the search for, or affirmation of, homosexual identity. My impressions from experiences as both participant in and facilitator of, safer-sex workshops during the last six years have led me to agree with these authors, and to think that the most urgent issues emotionally for many homosexuals relate to fear of being infected in each new relationship, to living with the threat of the illness or of death, and to identification with the danger to self and society. In prejudiced visions—especially those found in medical-epidemiological discourses—the homosexual oscillates between being victim and being villain, in the history of AIDS. How can one mobilize support and resources to overcome these images, to express and defeat those fears, without increasing the fear of being exposed? How can one break the solitude, silence, and secrets involved with being seropositive—or with having homosexual practices? How can one live with the fear that AIDS may appear and reveal one's sexual identity and secrets? And what, if this happens, can one do? For some, such risks may be as serious as being infected by HIV.

As suggested by Pollak (1993), AIDS brought to homosexuality the bursting of silence and the exposure of homosexual practices. The studies conducted on homosexual behaviors have already demystified what previously belonged to the realm of secrets and shadows. The media, especially in the beginning, seemed determined to transform homosexuality into a morbid "show" from which evil disseminated. Perlongher describes the media's treatment of homosexuality in those times as "crude descriptions of the vicissitudes of anal coitus, of the depth of penetration, the strength of fellatio, and the lethality of the kiss reached the living-room of families, complemented by information on the promiscuous people and their diabolic 'performances' " (Perlongher, 1987b). From such statements, a view was created in which every homosexual AIDS patient somehow deserved his fate, with death the logical consequence of the homosexual way of life.

How to live with prejudice, threat of discovery, and risk of infection may still be an issue for many men. There are known cases of men who, fearing exposure, preferred to die rather than to seek adequate medical treatment. How many still feel ashamed or frightened to buy condoms, believing such an act could expose their homosexual identity? There are growing numbers of family tragedies and destroyed marriages when one partner or relative hesitates, to the very last moment, to reveal his seropositivity—and often, in heterosexual marriage, his homosexuality?

Besides this sometimes threatening visibility, the logic of prevention embedded in the intervention actions of educational projects may be oppressive and provoke complex dilemmas; an example is the emphasis on a borderline between the "before" and the "after" of AIDS (Dannecker, 1991). The "before" of AIDS was the time when everything was permitted, when sex did not have rules and was free and guiltless; the "after" is a time when fear of infection prevails and one runs the risk of being alone, either because the negotiations about safer sex are not successful, or because sexual contacts may have been not as "good" as "before." With the advent of AIDS, the sexual act must be manipulated, and risk has to be considered, measured, even excluded, within the new parameters of healthy sex. Health and death are the two rhyming words that have come to guide homosexual pleasures.

Additionally, AIDS brings to homosexuality the new condition of being seropositive. It is no longer possible to deny the presence of seropositivity in the spaces of homoerotic encounters—saunas, parties, beaches, meetings with friends or boyfriends. The issue is omnipresent: how to live with this condition, be part of this reality and its difficult dimensions, knowing seropositivity can happen to anyone?

Indeed, seropositivity has many elements in common with homosexuality: silence, secrecy, the possibility of coming out, the unknown, solitude, threat of rejection, repression of self and of affection. Sedgwick (1990) suggests that, unlike many other stigmas—for example, those related to ethnic groups, which are revealed by visible characteristics—homosexuality (and seropositivity) can often be invisible, hidden, secret, dependent on revelation to become explicit. The fear of that revelation is twofold; he who makes the revelation often does not well understand what he is revealing, and he cannot know how his listener will react in face of the revealed mystery. As suggested by Pollak (1993), consideration of the family may illustrate this situation more radically. How many families discovered the homosexuality of a member only when his seropositivity was revealed? How many families hid a member's illness in order not to reveal his homosexual identity?

Seropositivity imposes the perspective of a new "coming out" for those who, after going through the process of recognizing themselves as homosexuals, now may also have to come out as seropositive (see Herdt, 1991). When this possibility materializes, the experiences of that first "coming out" may, according to Carricaburu and Pierret (1992), be decisive for this second passage. The previous affirmation may facilitate the confrontation with the stigmas imposed by AIDS, and may stimulate more constructive attitudes toward living with HIV.

Unlike other social groups affected by AIDS (for example, men with hemophilia, heterosexual men), homosexuals generally rapidly confronted the epidemic's challenges, including the positive processing of seropositivity—disconnecting it from the idea of illness by affirming that "being seropositive" did not mean "being ill," and that a "seropositive" was a "person equal to others" (Carricaburu and Pierret, 1992). Such attitudes helped to demystify seropositivity, stimulating a better quality of life.

The collective recent history of homosexuality is strongly marked by AIDS. This long familiarity with the epidemic—its representations, stigmas, pain, and grief—may facilitate living with HIV for the seropositive homosexuals within this wider collective. The capacity for collectively confronting the epidemic's challenges often resides in recognizing this, and it is here that solidarity emerges, in this sharing and participating, directly or indirectly, in a common history.

In the work of AIDS/NGOs and gay groups, safer-sex workshops have been among the most popular forms of meetings. The initial objective of these meetings was to increase the availability of information on safer sex. At first, these meetings stressed group communication exercises and other techniques of group dynamics, almost always with educational objectives, such as teaching techniques of safer sex that might preserve both pleasure and health.

Upon evaluation, these initial methodologies were questioned, as facilitators realized that participants were seeking not only to learn about safer sex but primarily to obtain tools for managing a daily life marked by doubt, uncertainty, threat, grief, and the other difficulties imposed by AIDS. Most attendees were searching for ways to escape from solitude, for opportunities to socialize individual dilemmas and confront oppression and fear often worsened by the epidemic.

Safer-sex workshops have increasingly changed from learning places into cultural reference and meeting points that facilitate new friendships, moments of leisure, information exchange on health, civil rights, arts, and so on, as well as places for teaching and learning. They provide opportunities to collectivize feelings and needs imposed by living with the epidemic and thus promote the solidarity of sharing and participating in problems and issues while coming to recognize these also are one's own. The meetings of the AIDS/NGOs and gay groups overlap with the places (such as bars, night-clubs, and saunas) where homosexuals have traditionally met, offering opportunities for meeting people and being with peers. In Rio de Janeiro, São Paulo, and other Brazilian cities, some organizations have gone so far as to set up "bars" or "night-clubs" in their own facilities; others organize sessions for viewing pornographic (and non-pornographic) films about homosexuality; still others offer drama workshops, gymnastics, or debates on current issues. These meetings represent a new development as, unlike commercial places, they are not aiming, generally, first at making a profit. This detail becomes important in a country like Brazil living with a longterm recession, since these initiatives widen the options of meeting places and, thus, socialization of low-income people whose economic exclusion makes access more difficult to cultural events and information (Parker and Terto, 1998).

Although still only partially articulated, the response of gay groups and, to an extent, the AIDS/NGOs reinforces the creation of new references and cultural symbols for homosexuality in Brazil. These include adoption of the rainbow (now an international gay symbol) at gay places and activities, organization of meetings around issues of safer sex and STDs, and production of videos, plays, and educational materials in which AIDS occupies an important position. Just as historical facts in Brazil, such as the political opening, the rebuilding of democracy, the reorganization of popular movements, and the liberalization of lifestyles redefined the cultural meanings of homosexuality at the end of the 1970s and beginning of the 1980s, AIDS constituted one of the most important historical facts for the redefinition of homosexual cultures and identities since the late 1980s in Brazil and many other countries (see Herdt and Boxer, 1991; Parker, 1994, 1999; Altman, 1989). To the old association of homosexuality with an "exotic," "forbidden," and "rule-less" sexuality based solely on physical pleasure, were added new meanings stressing solidarity, community, and citizenship, which must be considered in any understanding of male homosexuality in the 1990s.

AIDS is here to stay among homosexuals. Even were a vaccine discovered today, the consequences of the epidemic would be felt for a long time. Its impact among men who have sex with men is still difficult to evaluate, yet AIDS is now one of the most important factors in the construction of homoeroticism and homosexual subcultures throughout the world (see Altman, 1993; Parker, 1999). More than the affirmation of a homosexual identity, or the liberation of (homo)sexual desires, marking the activism of fifteen years ago, solidarity in response to AIDS may be a means to mobilize collectively and to find, or reinforce, solutions aiming at a better life for society as a whole.

Conclusion

In trying to understand how AIDS has affected homosexuality in Brazil, it is important to consider political, individual, and historical dimensions. In considering the characteristics of the epidemic and of male homosexuality in Brazil, I have come to agree with Edwards (1992) that research on the impact of AIDS on homosexuals leads also to understanding the impact homosexuals have on the epidemic's course. On the one hand, the growing numbers of homosexual men with HIV and AIDS show that homosexuals have been greatly affected by the epidemic. On the other, a historical perspective reveals the definitive influence homosexuals have had on society's responses to AIDS and in the construction of their own social representations about the epidemic and about themselves.

It becomes difficult to talk about these processes when considering only singular dimensions, since AIDS is not only a medical-epidemiological phenomenon but a social phenomenon with many effects, such as the complex political and social connections outlined in this article. According to McNeill (1989), epidemics are as important for historical and social change as are revolutions, wars, and discoveries. The diversity of effects considered here expresses the dynamism of the epidemic, which makes it impossible to draw conclusive analyses yet, since the epidemic continues to grow and its effects to change, amplified and moving in different directions in accordance with the resistances, vulnerabilities, responses, and oppositions resulting from personal, political, and social factors (Edwards, 1992). Thus, in this text I have considered factors as diverse as life histories, activism, historical episodes, the construction of individual identities, and efforts for prevention, as part of a complex process of historical change in which homosexual and seropositive identities have been shaped.

The effects of seropositivity not only within gay activism but also in social relations, family life, and the daily lives of individuals (not only of homosexuals) are issues that will require continued analysis as the epidemic grows not only in terms of the number of new cases, but also of the quantity of people visibly living with AIDS. In all likelihood, homosexuals will still constitute the majority of people visibly living with AIDS in Brazil for years to come. A series of issues concerning not only civil rights, legal recognition of homosexual marriages and inheritances, work, and social security, but also the construction and experience of sexuality and "otherness" should be added to the agenda for debates about a future that remains full of uncertainties for men who have sex with men.

References

Altman, D. (1989). "AIDS and the Reconceptualization of Homosexuality." In Altman, D. et al. (eds.), *Which Homosexuality?: Essays from the International Scientific Conference on Lesbian and Gay Studies*, 35–48. London: GMP Publishers.

———. (1993). "AIDS and the Discourses of Sexuality." In Connell, R. W., and Dowsett, G. W., (eds.), *Rethinking Sex*, 32–48. Philadelphia: Temple University Press.

———. (1994). *Power and Community: Organizational and Cultural Responses to AIDS*. London: Taylor and Francis.

Carricaburu, D., and Pierret, J. (1992). *Vie Quotidienne et Recompositions Identitaires autour de la Séropositivité*. Paris: CERMES.

Costa, J. F. (1992). *A Inocência e o Vício: Estudos sobre o Homoerotismo*. Rio de Janeiro: Relume-Dumará.

Daniel, H., and Míccolis, L. (1983). *Jacarés e Lobisomens—Dois Ensaios sobre a Homosexualidade*. Rio de Janeiro: Achiamé.

Daniel, H., and Parker, R. G. (1991). *AIDS: A Terceira Epidemia—Ensaios e Tentativas*. São Paulo: Iglu.

———. (1993). *Sexuality, Politics, and AIDS in Brazil*. London: Falmer Press.

Dannecker, M. (1991). *Der Homosexuelle Mann in Zeichen von AIDS*. Hamburg: Klein Verlag.

da Silva, C. C. (1993). *Triângulo Rosa: A Busca pela Cidadania dos Homossexuais*. Unpublished master's thesis. IFCS, Universidade Federal do Rio de Janeiro.

Edwards, T. (1992). "The AIDS Dialectics: Awareness, Identity, Death, and Sexual Politics." In Plummer, K. (ed.), *Modern Homosexualities*, 151–159. London: Routledge.

Fry, P. (1982). *Para Inglês Ver*. Rio de Janeiro: Zahar.

Fry, P. and MacRae, E. (1983). *O Que É Homosexualidade?* São Paulo: Brasiliense.

Harrad, D. (1995). "Estudos de Comportamento." Paper presented at the seminar Homossexualidades Brasileiras, Instituto de Medicina Social, Universidade do Estado do Rio de Janeiro.

Herdt, G. (1991). " 'Coming Out' as Rite of Passage: A Chicago Study." In Herdt, G. (ed.), *Gay Culture in America*, 29–67. Boston: Beacon Press.

Herdt, G., and Boxer, A. (1991). "Introduction: Culture, History, and Life Course of Gay Men." In Herdt, G. (ed.), *Gay Culture in America*, 1–28. Boston: Beacon Press.

MacRae, E. (1990). *A Construção da Igualdade: Identidade Sexual e Política no Brasil da Abertura*. Campinas: Unicamp.

McNeill, W. (1989). *Plagues and Peoples*. New York: Anchor Books.

Mott, L. (1997). *Homofobia: Violação dos Direitos Humanos de Gays, Lésbicas, e Travestis no Brasil*. San Francisco: Grupo Gay da Bahia/International Gay and Lesbian Human Rights Commission (IGLHRC).

Murray, S. (1992). "The 'Underdevelopment' of Modern/Gay Homosexuality in Meso-America." In Plummer, K. (ed.), *Modern Homosexualities*, 29–38. London: Routledge.

Parker, R. G. (1991). *Bodies, Pleasures, and Passions: Sexual Culture in Contemporary Brazil*. Boston: Beacon Press.

———. (1994). *A Construção da Solidariedade: AIDS, Sexualidade, e Política no Brasil*. Rio de Janeiro: Relume-Dumará.

———. (1999). *Beneath the Equator: Cultures of Desire, Male Homosexuality, and Emerging Gay Communities in Brazil*. New York and London: Routledge.

Parker, R. G., Mota, M., and Lourenço, R. (1994). "Sexo Entre Homens: Uma Pesquisa sobre a Consciência da AIDS e Comportamento Sexual no Brasil, 1989–1994." *Boletim ABIA Especial*, Associação Brasileira Interdisciplinar de AIDS.

Parker, R. G., and Terto Jr., V. (eds.). (1998). *Entre Homens: Homossexualidade e AIDS no Brasil*. Rio de Janeiro: ABIA.

Perlongher, N. (1987a). *O Negócio Do Michê: A Prostituição Viril*. São Paulo: Brasiliense.

———. (1987b). *O Que É AIDS?* São Paulo: Brasiliense.

Pollak, M. (1993). *Une Identité Blessée*. Paris: Métailié.

Sedgwick, E. K. (1990). *Epistemology of the Closet*. Berkeley and Los Angeles: University of California Press.

Seffner, F. (1995). "Homossexualidade e AIDS no Imaginário Social: Uma Possibilidade de Abordagem." Paper presented at the seminar Homossexualidades Brasileiras, Instituto de Medicina Social, Universidade do Estado do Rio de Janeiro.

Terto Jr., V. (1989). *No Escurinho do Cinema: Sociabilidade Orgiástica nas Tardes Cariocas*. Unpublished master's thesis. Department of Psychology, Pontifica Universidade Católica. Rio de Janeiro.

———. (1997). *Reinventando a Vida: Histórias sobre Homossexualidade e AIDS no Brasil*. Unpublished doctoral dissertation. Instituto de Medicina Social, Universidade do Estado do Rio de Janeiro.

Trevisan, J. S. (1986). *Devassos no Paraíso*. São Paulo: Max Limonad.

Watney, S. (1993). *Policing Desire: Pornography, AIDS and the Media*, 2d edition. MN: University of Minnesota Press.

Part Two

Sex, Gender, and Power

Chapter Four

Sexual Rights

Inventing a Concept, Mapping an International Practice

Rosalind P. Petchesky

"Sexual rights" is the newest kid on the block in international debates about the meanings and practices of human rights, especially women's human rights. That such a concept, and lively discussions about it, have finally surfaced in large international forums—in spite of or because of the pervasive climate of resurgent fundamentalisms in the world—surely in itself marks a historic achievement that feminist, and gay and lesbian, movements should proudly claim. Yet at this stage the concept is far from clear, not only among its staunch opponents but also among many advocates. It may be that "sexual rights" has become *both* a progressive wedge, opening up new space in the human rights lexicon for acknowledgement of diverse sexualities and their legitimate need for expression; *and* a kind of code that, like "reproductive rights," means different things to different speakers, depending on power position, sexual orientation, gender, nationality, and so on. Moreover, the risks, ambiguities, and potential misunderstandings of trying to negotiate sexuality through the arcane channels of international human rights procedures are troublesome. When it comes to sex, a chasm still separates the local and the global.

In what follows, I shall lay out some general reflections on the tenuous place where sexual rights discourse and politics currently hang suspended. First, I will briefly review recent developments in international conferences—particularly the world population conference in Cairo and the women's conference in Beijing, in 1994 and 1995, respectively—that have given birth to a still infantile (if not embryonic) sexual-rights language. Second, I will consider some difficulties in promoting a positive, or affirmative, concept of sexual rights, one that goes beyond the urgent but more acceptable struggle to combat the discriminations, abuses, and horrors committed against sexual minorities (including women who stray from dominant gender norms). The larger context for such difficulties, as I will show, is shared by all affirmative approaches to rights as goods, entitlements, and, ultimately, transformed social arrangements, rather than as solely defenses against discrimination or bodily harm. Third, I will outline some basic elements of what such an affirmative approach to sexual rights might involve, and its implications for social rights generally.[1] Finally, I will speculate about why even feminist, human rights, and other progressive groups have often been complicit in suppressing positive definitions of sexual rights, either actively or by omission; what factors in our ideological and political legacy contribute to this silence; what we have to lose from continuing this evasive or complicit practice; and what we have to gain from coming out in favor of sexual rights in a positive, liberatory sense.

Without going into details, let me review at least the outcomes of the recent United Nations conference debates that began to craft an incipient concept of sexual rights. Significantly, *no international instrument relevant to human rights, prior to 1993, makes any reference whatsoever to the forbidden "S" word* (other than "sex" as in biological sexes); that is, *prior to 1993 sexuality of any sort or manifestation is absent from international human rights discourse.* This may seem unremarkable when we consider the rigid division between public and private spheres that, as feminist critics have repeatedly pointed out, prevails in human rights implementation and enforcement mechanisms (Bunch, 1990; Cook, 1994; Copelon, 1994; Freedman and Isaacs, 1993; Romany, 1994). Yet, even if we confine human rights to the responsibilities of states, leaving out the responsibilities of other institutions or private persons, it must be said that, in fact, there has never been a sharp division between "private" and "public" in accepted human rights principles. Every major human rights document going back to the Universal Declaration of 1948 has much to say about the rights of persons in their private and personal lives: to marry and form a family, to express their beliefs and religion, to educate their children, to be respected in their privacy and homes, and so on—but nothing about expressing and being secure in their sexuality. Moreover, neither do any women's conference declarations prior to 1992 refer to women's sexuality, much less to sexual rights—not the Women's Convention (Convention on the Elimination of All Forms of Discrimination Against Women, 1981) nor the Nairobi Forward-Looking Strategies (1985), which refer to sexual equality and women's right to control over their fertility, but not to sexual freedom or the rights of lesbians. In other words, in most human rights discourse, until very recently, sexual life is acknowledged only implicitly, and then confined within the bounds of heterosexual marriage and repro-duction (see Cook, 1995; Copelon and Hernandez, 1994).[2]

A major turning point came in 1993, with the World Conference on Human Rights in Vienna, where, thanks to the concerted efforts of a well-organized women's lobby for human rights, the Declaration and Programme of Action called on states to eliminate "gender based violence and all forms of sexual harassment and exploitation," includ-ing trafficking in women, "systematic rape, sexual slavery, and forced pregnancy" (paragraphs 18 and 38). The Declaration on the Elimi-nation of Violence Against Women, passed by the United Nations General Assembly that same year, contains even more explicit con-demnation of various forms of "physical, sexual, and psychological violence against women" (paragraph 2) and makes it clear—thanks again to the work of feminist international legal scholars—that this prohibition is not something new but rather stems directly from time-honored principles embedded in international human rights law. These include, among others, the rights to life, liberty, and security of the person (Universal Declaration, Article 3; European Convention on Human Rights, Article 2); to the inviolability of the person and of physical and mental integrity (African Charter on Human and Peo-ples' Rights, Articles 4 and 6; American Convention on Human Rights, Article 5); and to freedom from torture and cruel and inhuman punishment (Cook, 1995). Indeed, feminist scholars have established a clear link between torture and rape or other forms of sexual vio-lence, whether in the context of war or that of domestic relations (Copelon, 1994).

The Vienna Declaration and the Declaration on Violence Against Women were important not only because they gained recognition of sexual violence as a human rights violation but also because they fi-nally initiated "the sexual" into human rights language. Yet not until the International Conference on Population and Development (ICPD), in Cairo in 1994, would sexuality begin to sneak into inter-national documents as something positive rather than violent, abu-sive—or sanctified—and hidden within heterosexual marriage and childbearing. As Yasmin Tambiah puts it, "the Cairo Document is indisputably one of the most progressive statements acknowledging sexual activity as a positive aspect of human society to emerge recently through global consensus" (Tambiah, 1995). Many government delegates at the Cairo conference (particularly those from Islamic or Catholic countries where fundamentalists have great political influence) made no secret of their complete aversion to letting the bad "S" word appear anywhere in the ICPD Programme of Action; it remained bracketed until nearly the final hour. Yet, in the document's final version, references to "sex" and "sexuality" appear numerous times, and for the first time in any international legal instrument, the ICPD Programme explicitly includes "sexual health" (if not sexual pleasure) in the array of rights that population and development programs should protect. Chapter 7 of the document adopts the World Health Organization's official definition of "sexual health" as an integral part of reproductive health, requiring "that people are able to have a satisfying and safe sex life" as well as to decide "if, when, and how often" to reproduce. It defines the purpose of sexual health as "the enhancement of life and personal relations, and not merely counseling and care related to reproduction and sexually transmitted diseases" (paragraph 7.1).

There is little doubt that the concerns of many delegations, especially from sub-Saharan Africa, about the devastating health and social consequences of HIV/AIDS played a crucial role in bringing sexuality into the ICPD document—a role at least as important as that of the women's human rights coalition in foregrounding women as victims of sexual violence. Nonetheless, the extent to which "a satisfying and safe sex life" as an affirmative, not only a disease-preventive, goal appears in the Programme is surprising. One doesn't want to overstate this; nowhere did freedom of sexual expression and orientation gain recognition as a human right, at the Cairo conference or anyplace since. Yet, while there is no explicit reference to sexual rights for gays, lesbians, or unmarried persons (or anyone else, for that matter), neither does paragraph 7.2 expressly limit its principle of self-determination, safety, and satisfaction in sexual life to heterosexuals, married couples, or adults (Copelon and Petchesky, 1995). Indeed, other provisions in chapter 7 refer to "the limited power many women and girls have over their sexual and reproductive lives" and urge governments to provide adolescents a full array of sexual and reproductive health services and education "to enable them to deal in a positive and responsible way with their sexuality." While "voluntary absti-nence" is offered as one means toward the goal of men "[sharing] responsibility with women in matters of sexuality and reproduction," so too are condoms (that nefarious and finally unbracketed "C" word) (paragraphs 7.3, 7.41, 7.44, 7.45, and 8.31). Finally—and most con-troversially, as it turned out—signatory governments to the ICPD Programme pledge in chapter 5 that their laws and policies will take into account the "plurality of [family] forms" existing in most societies (paragraphs 5.1 and 5.2).

The Platform for Action produced by the Fourth World Women's Conference, in Beijing in 1995, went further toward formulating a concept of sexual rights as an international human rights principle. There, a complicated negotiation process involving delegates, the Vatican-led fundamentalists, some wily chairs, and the women's NGO coalition hammered out the following historic paragraph:

The human rights of women include their right to have control over and decide freely and responsibly on matters related to their sexuality, including sexual and reproductive health, free of coercion, discrimination and violence. Equal relationships between women and men in matters of sexual relations and reproduction, including full respect for the integrity of the person, re-quire mutual respect, consent and shared responsibility for sexual behavior and its consequences. (paragraph 96)

This text is remarkable for both its utterances and its silences, what it makes explicit in the repertoire of international declarations (which are nonbinding but morally incumbent on their signatories) and what it still leaves hidden. Notice that for the first time, women are ac-knowledged as sexual as well as reproductive beings, with human rights to decide freely about their sexuality without any express qual-ification regarding age, marital status, or sexual orientation. But notice too that the original formulation of the paragraph, which had been bracketed in the draft, stated *not* "the human rights of women" but "the sexual rights of women." In the final version of the Platform, the phrase "sexual rights" disappears altogether; the phrase "sexual ori-entation" (much less "lesbian" or "gay") never even made it into the draft, whereas "reproductive rights"—"the capability to reproduce and the freedom to decide if, when and how often to do so"—is now codified, through both Cairo and Beijing, in human rights treaty language.[3] Moreover, since the phrase "respect for the integrity of the person" was introduced to replace any reference to "bodily integrity" or the body in any form (which some feminists feared would be applied to the fetus), nowhere in the Beijing Platform do sexualized female bodies—or non-heterosexual bodies, claiming pleasures rather than fending off abuses—appear.

Of course, this absence is the outcome of a complex drama in the halls of the United Nations. In that drama the fine points of language become a critical terrain for the contestation of power—and of the meanings of sexuality—through endless spirals of domination, resistance, and reconstitution of discourse (Petchesky, 1993, 1997). A formidable coalition of feminist nongovernmental organizations (NGOs) from both South and North working tirelessly at the Cairo and Beijing conferences was able to stake new ground on this terrain, in the face of much stronger forces among fundamentalists and the more conservative population groups and governments. In Cairo, the feminist coalition had succeeded in transforming the discourse of "reproductive rights" from a Westernist code for abortion into an international United Nations language denoting women's human right to self-determination over their fertility, motherhood, and, to a limited degree, sexuality. It was inevitable that this victory would call forth a backlash, in the immediate aftermath of the ICPD, revealing where the hard lines would be drawn. For there is no doubt that underneath the aversion to sexual rights lurk taboos against homosexuality, bisexuality, and alternative family forms. Listen to two typical reservations to the final ICPD Programme of Action, registered by dissenting delegations. Holy See: "With reference to the term 'couples and individuals,' the Holy See reserves its position with the understanding that this term is to mean *married couples and the individual man and woman who constitute the couple*." Egypt: "Our delegation called for the deletion of the word 'individuals' since it has always been our understanding that all the questions dealt with by the Programme of Action . . . relate to harmonious relations between couples united by the bond of marriage in the context of . . . the family as the primary cell of society" (United Nations, 1994, 144–46).

In the prelude to Beijing, this drift continued. Having basically lost the verbal contest in Cairo, including on the question of "diverse family forms," the Vatican-led fundamentalist alliance conducted a concerted media campaign, in the period leading up to the Beijing Women's Conference, designed to taint the concepts of "reproductive and sexual rights" with the labels of "individualism," "Western feminism," and lesbianism. This campaign not only opposed the language of "reproductive rights" and "diverse family forms" but, for a time, also succeeded in bracketing all references to the word "gender"! The reason for this puzzling maneuver, as feminists involved in the Third Preparatory Meeting learned, was that Vatican representatives had obtained a women's studies course packet from the United States containing readings that not only explained gender as a social construct (rather than a biological given) but also evoked the possibility of changing genders, multiple genders, and so on; hence the Vatican delegation's insistence that "sex," not "gender," should be the official terminology.

In the actual Beijing Women's Conference, the fundamentalist campaign against "gender" and "sexual rights" fronted as a crusade on behalf of "parental rights," but its real targets were clearly lesbian sexuality and the sexuality of all unmarried adolescents. A flier distributed by a group of North American Vatican-aligned women called Coalition for Women and the Family made perfectly plain the homophobia that Holy See delegates were far too politic to display in official United Nations sessions. Entitled "Sexual Rights and Sexual Orientation—What do these words really mean?" the flier associates "these words" with not only homosexuality, lesbianism, and sexual relationships outside marriage and among adolescents, but also "pedophilia," "prostitution," "incest," and "adultery." And it engages in gay-baiting and fear-mongering (for example, with the statement "Homosexuals have claimed protection for behaviors which everyone knows spread HIV/AIDS"). Yet the fundamentalist position went deeper even than issues of sexual and bodily self-determination for women and gays, challenging the ethical and epistemological basis of claims to such rights. In his *Evangelium Vitae* encyclical—released to the media to coincide precisely with the March Preparatory Committee Meeting—the pope condemns ideas and practices asserting reproductive and sexual autonomy by associating them with "a hedonistic mentality unwilling to accept responsibility in matters of sexuality" and "a self-centered concept of freedom" (Catholics for a Free Choice, 1995; *Evangelium Vitae*, 1995).

But the Vatican alone cannot be blamed for the ambiguity that remains in the Beijing Platform's sexual rights formula. In a world-historical moment of religious patriarchal revivalism, accusations of "selfishness" and admonitions to self-sacrifice directed toward women have a powerful appeal. In such a climate, liberal groups also become susceptible to the backlash and begin to retreat or curb their demands. The United States delegation in Beijing, for example, made up mostly of women Democrats allied with the Clinton administration and very nervous about the power of right-wing conservatives back home, tempered its usual support for reproductive and women's rights by submitting an interpretive statement during the deliberations on paragraph 96 (cited earlier). In its statement, the United States emphasized three different times the phrases "relationships *between women and men*" and "freedom from coercion, discrimination and violence," thus seeming to deflect from any possible interpretation that would highlight lesbian identity or women's right to sexual pleasure.[4]

In the face of not just evasion but outright antagonism and "a sexphobic right wing that drew its strength from a multi-religious base" (Tambiah, 1996), women's groups from around the world involved in the official Beijing conference found it necessary to compromise on any affirmative, more controversial formulation of sexual rights. In March 1995, a petition signed by thousands of women and groups from sixty countries in all the world's regions had been presented to Gertrude Mongella, conference secretary-general, calling upon member states "to recognize the right to determine one's sexual identity; the right to control one's own body, particularly in establishing intimate relationships; and the right to choose if, when, and with whom to bear or raise children as fundamental components of the human rights of all women regardless of sexual orientation." Given the rancorous climate of the late-night deliberations on the final wording of paragraph 96, however, women's groups and their government allies found it difficult if not impossible to argue for such explicitly feminist and affirmative values.[5]

But why? Why is it so much easier to assert sexual freedom in a negative than in an affirmative, emancipatory sense; to gain consensus for the right not to be abused, exploited, raped, trafficked, or mutilated in one's body, but not the right to fully enjoy one's body? Aside from tactical positions and defenses against overt homophobia, is there a larger social, political, and economic context, as well as a particular ideological baggage, making such an assertive approach remain elusive in this historical moment? Before attempting to answer these questions, let me emphasize how important is the ground that feminist organizations, especially in the South, have gained toward recognition of reproductive and sexual rights as human rights. Women's and gay rights movements in countries where the Catholic Church is powerful—the Philippines, Nigeria, Brazil, Mexico, Peru, and elsewhere in Latin America—have struggled (still unsuccessfully, in most cases) to legalize abortion, reduce maternal mortality, and educate about safer sex and condom use. In Bangladesh, according to Sajeda Amin and Sara Hossain (1995), women's organizations have publically countered brutal attacks on women accused by Islamic religious tribunals of transgressing sexual norms. In Egypt, Sudan, Somalia, Kenya, and Nigeria, campaigns by women's groups against female genital mutilation have focused simultaneously on the procedure's erosion of women's sexual pleasure and on its severe risks to women's health (Toubia, 1995; Tambiah, 1995).

These efforts nourished the forcefulness of the women's coalitions in Vienna, Cairo, and Beijing, and their success in merging the language of sexual and reproductive health with the language of women's human rights. The synthesis thus created has in turn re-articulated a feminist ethics of bodily integrity and personhood that permeates the Cairo and Beijing documents and directly challenges the moral arsenal of Catholic, Jewish, and Islamic fundamentalists. This ethics postulates not only that women must be free from abuse and violation in their bodies (including their fertility and sexuality), but also that they must be treated as principal actors and decision makers, as the ends and not the means of population, health, and development programs. Moreover, through this ethics, this principle applies not only to states and their agents but to every level where power operates—in the home, the clinic, the workplace, the church, synagogue, or mosque, and the community (Corrêa and Petchesky, 1994; Corrêa, 1994; Sen and Snow, 1994).

Yet there is something disturbing in the way this shift to a feminist ethic of self-determination over our bodies, which has indisputably become a shared discourse across South and North, has opened only through negations, denials, and litanies on violence and abuse behind which the claims to pleasure remain ever silent. Of course human rights language, especially with second and third-generation rights, is supposed to embody affirmative entitlements and not just protections from abuse or discrimination; they are two sides of a coin (I cannot enjoy my sexual body if I am subjected to constant fear of battering or unwanted pregnancy) (Heise, 1995; Copelon, 1994; Copelon and Petchesky, 1995). Still, campaigns around women's human rights have generally gained widest attention when parading the worst horrors (genital mutilation, mass rape as a weapon of war, forced abortion or sterilization, sexual trafficking, murder of women for sexual or gender "deviance"); they therefore capitalize on the image of women as victims.[6] Given this tendency in feminist human rights discourse, it is no accident that in both the health and the human rights sections of the Beijing Platform, the specter of sexualized bodies claiming pleasures lurked *behind* the debates, present only in the absence of "bodies" and "sexual rights" in the final text. And this "victim"-izing tendency is troubling to the extent that it evades, or even mirrors, fundamentalist patriarchal images of women as weak and vulnerable.

To be sure, the problem with such negative constructions pervades human rights discourse in general. Historically, the human rights violations that receive the most attention and have the greatest possibility of enforcement have always been those involving blatant discrimination or physical abuse, the paradigm situations being those of torture victims and mistreated political prisoners. It is much more difficult to achieve anything but lip service from governments to their treaty commitments under the International Covenant on Economic, Social, and Cultural Rights (ICESCR), which includes important provisions subsequently incorporated in the Cairo and Beijing documents. For example, Article 12 of the ICESCR recognizes "the right of everyone to the enjoyment of the highest attainable standard of physical and mental health," now a major underpinning of the principles of reproductive and sexual health rights. But framing health in affirmative human rights terms means "conceptualizing [it] as a social good" basic to human dignity and well being "and not solely a medical, technical, or economic problem" (Leary, 1994). And this implies major obligations and redirection of resources on the part of governments, which must take positive action to assure that decent health care becomes a legitimate entitlement and accessible reality for all people under their jurisdiction; that is, they must create the necessary social conditions for health to become a social right. If very few societies in a world now dominated by capitalist markets take this view (rather than the view of health care as a private commodity), is it surprising that only one country, South Africa, has a constitution that recognizes the right to freedom of sexual orientation?

I do not wish to be misunderstood here. The rape, forced marriage, forced slavery, mutilation, and other forms of sexual violence imposed on thousands of women as part of the Rwandan genocide is only the most shocking recent example of a pattern of "hatreds" (to use Zillah Eisenstein's word) that intersects almost everywhere with racial and national antagonisms (Eisenstein, 1996; Human Rights Watch, 1996; Center for Women's Global Leadership, 1996; Rosenbloom, 1995). Less dramatic but as insidious in the long run is the criminalization of lesbianism in many countries, and mounting pressure from conservatives for enforcement of criminal bans in some of these.[7] My intention is not to deny or diminish the magnitude of such atrocities against women and sexual minorities. Rather, I am arguing that focusing on such cases—however horrifying and important in bringing media attention to the legitimacy of sexual rights as human rights—at best gets us to the level of liberal tolerance. The negative, exclusionary approach to rights, sometimes expressed as the right to "privacy" or to be "let alone" in one's choices and desires, can never in itself help construct an *alternative vision* or lead to fundamental structural, social, and cultural transformations. Even the feminist slogan "my body is my own," while rhetorically powerful, may be perfectly compatible with the hegemonic global market, insofar as it demands freedom from abuse but not from the economic conditions that compel a woman to sell her body or its sexual or reproductive capacities (Pateman, 1988; Petchesky, 1995).

What, then, would an alternative, positive vision of sexual rights look like? I would suggest it contains two integral and interlocked components: a set of *ethical principles* (expressing the substance, or ultimate ends, of sexual rights), and a wide range of *enabling conditions* without which those ends could not be achieved (Corrêa and Petchesky, 1994). These ethical principles include sexual diversity, habitational diversity ("diverse family forms"), health, decision-making autonomy (personhood), and gender equality. *Sexual diversity,* or "multisexualism," implies commitment to the principle that diverse types of sexual expression (not only the heterosexual or conjugal) are not only tolerable but beneficial to a just, humane, culturally pluralistic society. This principle places optimum value on the ethical goods of caring, affection, support, and mutually consensual erotic stimulation, assuming that the particular forms or relationships expressing these, whether heterosexual, homosexual, or bisexual, are secondary to the importance of a cultural climate that encourages their expression. (I am assuming a broad definition of "consent" that would preclude adult-child incest and other sexual relations between persons in grossly different power positions, such as prison guards and inmates, or doctors and patients.) A wealth of ethnographic and historical examples of such diversity existing in numerous societies and cultures is certainly available from the rich scholarship of gay and lesbian (or queer) studies of the past decade.[8] One may surmise that, from a broad cross-cultural and historical perspective, conjugal heterosexuality is far from a universal practice, and argue that rights, while not governed by social and cultural practices, ought at least to take their diversity into account.

A second, closely related principle, I am calling *habitational diversity* to separate it from procreation, which it may but does not necessarily involve. This principle has a precedent in the ICPD Programme of Action's repeated recognition of "diverse family forms," which created such havoc among the Vatican and its fundamentalist allies. While specifically mentioning only female-headed households, the Cairo document acknowledges that people cohabit, raise children, and sustain affective relations in many types of arrangements across the world's societies and cultures; implies that the patriarchal, conjugal, heterosexual family is neither exclusive nor inherently superior; and suggests that all sorts of families or cohabiting groups, regardless of structure, are "entitled to receive comprehensive protection and support" from the state (ICPD, paragraph 5.1). Probably the fundamentalists' fears that this language would sanction gay and lesbian families and marriages say more about the fundamentalists than about the intentions of member states. Nonetheless, the recognition of "diverse family forms" in the ICPD Programme does put the "right to marry and found a family," hallowed in major human rights instruments, in a rather new light.

The third ethical principle is that of *health*, and it too has already received international human rights codification. When we combine "the right of everyone to the enjoyment of the highest attainable standard of physical and mental health" with the recognition, in the Cairo document, that "sexual health" is part of reproductive rights and involves a "satisfying" as well as "safe" sexual life, we are approaching something that starts to look like *pleasure as a positive good*. Of course, the link to reproduction limits the scope, but not if the principle is taken in conjunction with sexual and habitational diversity. The point is that there is already some basis in existing international agreements for asserting the right to sexual pleasure as part of basic health and well-being necessary to human life—a concept recognized in several major world religions (including Islam and Judaism) as well as many traditional cultures.[9]

Fourth is the principle of *autonomy*, or *personhood*, implying the right of individuals—children and youth as well as adults—to make their own decisions in matters affecting their bodies and health. The principle is expressed eloquently in the pre-Beijing petition cited earlier ("Put Sexuality on the Agenda at the World Conference on Women"), as "the right to determine one's sexual identity; the right to control one's own body, particularly in establishing intimate relationships . . ." Clearly this principle is rooted in basic concepts of liberty and democracy, and is fundamental to citizenship (or pre-citizenship[10]) rights. In other words, so-called "civil and political rights" and "economic, social, and cultural rights" are, as feminist and other human rights advocates have stressed so often, interdependent and indivisible (Sen, 1990; Human Rights Watch, 1996; Copelon and Petchesky, 1995). For how can one act responsibly as a citizen and as a member of kin group and community if one's body and sexuality are defined and controlled by others—by husband, parents, religious authorities, or the state?

But, especially in the domain of sexual rights, it becomes clear the autonomy or personhood principle is inseparable from that of *gender equality*, when we recall the thousands of ways in all societies that the law of sexual norms is infused with a gender code as well as a family code. Yasmin Tambiah, in her splendid analysis of "Sexuality and Human Rights," encapsulates the inequities in the girl child's situation in so many societies, the "contradictory messages" that cripple the development of her sexuality:

She is instructed to devalue her own body lest she be responsible for inciting unwarranted male attention. Simultaneously she is expected to cultivate the ability to hold male attention as a desireable wife. She is kept ignorant about her body because it is alleged that the less she knows about it, the less likely she is to explore her sexuality and therefore compromise her virginity. At the same time, however, she is expected to develop a healthy and knowledgeable attitude toward motherhood. (Tambiah, 1995, 374)

Tambiah's observation that the girl child is thus "compelled into heterosexuality, being denied the opportunity to develop an understanding of her sexuality and eventually to exercise an informed, autonomous choice," confirms some of the findings of the International Reproductive Rights Research Action Group (IRRRAG) in a recent study in seven countries in Africa, Asia, the Americas, and the Middle East.[11] Discouragingly, we found that older generations of women, denied other channels of authority or outlets for self-assertion, are even more likely than men in many communities to police the boundaries of other women's (and their own daughters') sexual behavior. As is well known, women may acquire a certain privileged status or respectability from upholding traditional practices and codes of honor.[12] Likewise, Tambiah's description of women's *normative* condition, heterosexual marriage, as fraught with dangers, both physical and social, and of the need to constantly walk a fine line with regard to sexuality, echoes the findings of our researchers. In one country study after another, we found women making "trade-offs," negotiating their sexual pleasure and autonomy in exchange for other gains. For example, in the Philippines, Mexico, and Egypt women accept unwanted marital sex in exchange for husbands' cooperation in housework, or to stave off quarrels or domestic violence. In Egypt women adapt to female genital mutilation, or to a wedding night defloration ritual they find painful and humiliating, to secure public respectability and the freedom to come and go.[13] In Brazil fear of domestic violence limits the physical and sexual mobility of rural women, while fear of pregnancy and job loss keeps domestic workers effectively celibate. And the majority of women we interviewed everywhere still believe that to express a need for sexual satisfaction, much less entitlement to it, will bring them shame.

Even as we encountered these sad and more familiar examples of sexual self-denial, however, IRRRAG's research also disclosed some voices of poor women, across diverse cultures and situations, who articulated an affirmative sense of entitlement to sexual pleasure as women. Sometimes this is vicarious, as with mothers who begin to identify with their daughters and seek sexual autonomy and pleasure for and through them, giving the trade-off strategy an intergenerational form. This was particularly true of working-class Brazilian housewives who rejected for their daughters the rigid virginity codes ingrained in themselves as young girls. My favorite respondent in our study was the São Paulo mother who told her daughter, "You have to obey your mother and be a good girl. Even if you have sex, do it carefully, use a condom. Know what you are doing . . . because, if afterwards you have a child, who will take care of your children? There are so many ways to avoid it . . ." While obviously reflecting fear of the widespread risk of HIV/AIDS and other STDs in urban Brazil, such mothers are also taking the traditional definition of "good girl" and turning it upside down (Portella et al., 1998).

In other examples, affirmative expressions of sexual entitlement among grassroots women may be indirect—for example, the *maquilladora* worker from Sonora, Mexico, who complained women "don't have the chance to like [sex]" because men are always aggressive and overbearing and "only care for their own satisfaction" (Ortiz-Ortega et al., 1998). Elsewhere they are more direct, such as the nineteen-year-old woman in northern Nigeria who defiantly announced, "Whenever I feel like sleeping with my boyfriend, I go to him" (Osakue and Martin-Hilber, 1998), or the forty-year-old farm worker from the Sertão region of Brazil, who certified that concepts of sexual freedom are not solely the property of urban middle-class activists: "It's a matter of choice. If someone feels better with a man, she should keep to him . . . If I like a woman, it's my business. I've got to think of myself, not of what others may say . . . Everyone has the right to choose what is right for herself" (Portella et al., 1998).

Yet these affirmative sexual claims by grassroots women have to be seen as, at present, more wishes or aspirations than concrete realities. For most women, their realization in practice depends on the crucial component of sexual rights (mentioned earlier), *enabling conditions*. Indeed, the five ethical principles I have sketched will remain useless abstractions, particularly given the huge cutbacks and privatization of social services that women in all seven IRRRAG countries, and throughout the world, are facing, without global economic, social, and structural changes. How is decision-making autonomy over sexuality possible without full information about safer sex, sexuality, one's body, contraceptive methods, and ways to avoid STDs? How is sexual health possible without access to preventive, caring, and quality services and methods? How is habitational diversity possible without adequately commodious housing, a place and space to be intimate? More profoundly, how are sexual diversity and gender equality possible without a cultural revolution in how societies, media, and institutions envision "women" and "men"? In other words, if we ask (in human rights lingo) what would be the minimal criteria for developing indicators whereby United Nations agencies and governments could establish standards for measuring compliance with sexual rights principles, we begin to see that an affirmative approach to sexual rights opens enormous transformational visions that would affect men as well as women, all of society and not only its sexual minorities.

But if this is the case, why have many progressive organizations, including women's and human rights groups, been so tentative about mobilizing behind an affirmative and comprehensive sexual rights program? Why, more particularly, are so many of us complicit in maintaining the invisibility of sex as pleasure? There are many reasons, some hidden and some obvious, and no space here to explore them at length. Short of outright homophobia (which unfortunately still contaminates many organizations), they involve a certain ideological baggage—the legacy of the left and its economistic biases and suspicions of "bourgeois individualism," the legacy of nationalism and its suspicions of Western cultural imperialism, the legacy of the Foucauldian post-modernism that both "discovered" and inscribed the agentic sexual self as an illusion of the European Enlightenment. There is also the political contradiction built into the feminist and gay rights movements to the extent that both seek at the same time to transform societies and to find "a place at the table." Aspiring to influence and power in the public realm—including power over the terms of human rights rhetoric—always contains risks of compromise and co-optation, risks that necessarily contributed to the ambiguities over the meanings of "sexual rights" in the final Beijing document. What we can say is this: "the body" evokes the fetal body for some and women's sexualized body, including the lesbian body, for others; either way, it remains dangerous and commands silence. Sexual self-determination and sexual rights imply both the negative freedom against unwanted intrusions, violations, and abuses, and the positive capacity to seek and experience pleasures in a variety of ways and situations, including (for women) modes without a man. But the latter concept is still too dangerous for affirmative reiteration among many women's movements.

While I am convinced that affirmative constructions of rights need more of our attention, as both intellectuals and activists, the "liberatory" approach to sexual rights poses its own dilemmas.

First, am I overly dichotomizing the "pleasure" and "danger" sides of sexuality and thus ignoring the dialectical way the affirmative and negative dimensions of rights intertwine? Amartya Sen, addressing the more general concept of freedom, makes a powerful argument that "the social commitment to individual freedom has to be concerned with both positive and negative freedoms, and with their extensive interconnections" (Sen, 1990, 50). Not only does a person's right to fully develop and enjoy her body and her erotic and emotional capacities depend on freedom from abuse and violence, and on having the necessary enabling conditions and material resources, as discussed earlier; it may also be that awareness of affirmative sexual rights comes as a result of experiencing their violation.[14] An interesting life trajectory discovered by IRRRAG researchers in several countries was one in which a woman, beaten or systematically subjected to unwanted sex by her husband over many years, had finally resisted effectively (sometimes wielding a knife!), after which she gained a sense of empowerment that led to new forms of independent earning, a new relationship, or both.

Second, as an umbrella category attempting to be inclusive and universal, sexual rights can become a totalizing language that actually excludes and obscures. The now-mainstreamed elision of the phrase "sexual and reproductive rights" among feminist reproductive health advocates too often buries the sexual, folding it discreetly into marital/heterosexual and childbearing relations (see IPPF, 1996; Cook, 1995). Nowhere do any existing human rights instruments, including the Cairo and Beijing documents, articulate either freedom of sexual orientation or diverse sexualities; thus, to the extent that "sexual rights" continues to rely on interpretations of these instruments, or to collapse the "sexual" into the "reproductive," the specific rights and situations of lesbians, bisexual women, and a whole range of culturally specific sexual minorities may remain invisible. Thus we must still ask how we may create a general rights framework that also addresses these specificities.[15] Moreover, reticence about sexual practices and their diversity may affect not only human rights interpretation but also the accuracy of field research. Surely it says more about the sensitivities of IRRRAG's researchers than about the practices of our respondents that in almost none of our seven studies is lesbian sexuality to be found.

At the same time, it is crucial to recognize that these silences I find disturbing are based as much on strategic calculation as on deep inner conflict. In many countries and communities still, to speak openly of women's right to varied sexual pleasures is to invite the closing of one's organization, ostracism of its members, verbal and physical attacks, even death. The spiral of resistance is, as always, constrained by power; and these power dynamics are reproduced in the soul of each of us, however radical our vision. In this political context, to begin to speak of sexual rights, even tentatively, is a big step. In the research context, to begin to map out women's often compromising strategies for negotiating sexual entitlements can help us to see which conditions must change before we can empower the women we interview, and ourselves, to reach for strategies more daring.

Acknowledgments

For much of the thinking in this paper (though not for its flaws), I gratefully acknowledge stimulating discussions with Roxanna Carrillo, Susanna Fried, Claudia Hinojosa, Rachel Kyte, Ilana Lansberg-Lewis, Adriana Ortiz-Ortega, Rachel Rosenbloom, Yasmin Tambiah, the New Visions Faculty Seminar on Human Rights at Hunter College, and most especially the ideas and support of Rhonda Copelon.

Notes

1. Some of this analysis is drawn from a previous article I wrote with Sonia Corrêa (Corrêa and Petchesky, 1994).

2. On one level, this should not be surprising. Despite Foucault's (Eurocentric) insistence on characterizing modernity by its incessant preoccupation with sex talk, in fact we know how consistently such talk, even in the West, has been veiled, ambivalent, guilt laden, or scandal ridden. Only at the end of the twentieth century and the threshold of the new millennium have international relations become, largely as a result of the global HIV/ AIDS pandemic, a domain where sexuality can be somewhat openly discussed. (See Parker and Gagnon, 1995, especially the editors' introduction and article by Altman, and Foucault, 1978.)

3. Both the ICPD Programme (paragraph 7.2) and the Beijing Platform (paragraph 95) define "reproductive rights" as "[resting] on the recognition of the basic right of all couples and individuals to decide freely and responsibly the number, spacing, and timing of their children and to have the information and means to do so, and the right to attain the highest standard of sexual and reproductive health. It also includes their right to make decisions concerning reproduction free of discrimination, coercion, and violence, as expressed in human rights documents."

4. Thanks to Rhonda Copelon for providing a copy of this statement (dated September 14, 1995, submitted to the Main Committee of the FWWC in Beijing).

5. See Rosenbloom, 1995, Appendix A, for the full text of the petition. While I attended some earlier sessions of the official conference, I was not present at the meeting described. Many thanks to Roxanna Carillo, Rhonda Copelon, Rachel Kyte, and Ilana Landsberg-Lewis for sharing impressions of this historic moment.

6. This emphasis is very much present in two otherwise excellent and invaluable publications that offer chilling testimonies of the kinds of sexual abuse and violence that brutalize women (and gay men) throughout the world (see Center for Women's Global Leadership, 1996, and Rosenbloom, 1995).

7. For the case of recent anti-gay and anti-lesbian legislation and campaigns by fundamentalists in Sri Lanka, see Tambiah, 1996. According to the International Gay and Lesbian Human Rights Commission, eighty-six countries outlaw gay male homosexuality, compared to forty-four that criminalize lesbianism; clearly, lesbianism is seen as less of a threat, but only because of its "social invisibility" and the denial by some lawmakers that it even exists. (Rosenbloom, 1995:xiii.)

8. For just a few examples, see Parker and Gagnon, 1995, especially articles by Lützen, Herdt and Boxer, Tan, Lancaster, Zalduondo and Bernard, and Weeks; and the present volume, especially articles by Dowsett, Oetomo, and Terto.

9. Aihwa Ong (1994) notes that the *kampung* women she interviewed in Malaysia—apparently more influenced by *adat*, or village tradition, than by contemporary fundamentalist versions of Sharia'a law—considered sex "essential to good health and only viewed negatively when indulged in excessively or with an unsuitable partner."

10. In the case of children or immigrants.

11. See *Negotiating Reproductive Rights: Women's Perspectives across Countries and Cultures* (London: Zed Press, ed. R. Petchesky and K. Judd, 1998). IRRRAG's interdisciplinary research teams—made up of social science researchers, women's health movement and human rights activists, and health providers—carried out intensive qualitative research among low-income urban and rural women in Brazil, Egypt, Malaysia, Mexico, Nigeria,

the Philippines, and the United States in 1993 and 1994. The purpose was to find out the circumstances and areas in which such women—varying in age, marital status, ethnicity, religion, and occupation—begin to develop a sense of entitlement and self-determination around sexual and reproductive decision making.

12. In Nigeria, for example, we repeatedly observed how older rural and urban market women maintained and elevated their status in the community by enforcing traditional practices such as widowhood rites and female genital mutilation. In Egypt, we found that mothers were more likely than fathers to want to enforce the *baladi dokhla*, or wedding night ritual proving virginity, and to control their daughters' choice of marriage partner; apparently these are arenas where they felt they could maintain some kind of authority in the household. In several countries, mothers were unwilling to impart sexual knowledge to daughters prior to their marriage, for fear of "opening their eyes" and risking family dishonor.

13. Ironically, men interviewed in Egypt see this ritual as an "invasion of privacy"; only women feel compelled to trade bodily integrity for economic and civil rights that legally belong to them. See Aida Seif El Dawla, Amal Abdel Hadi, and Nadia Abdel Wahab, "Women's Wit Over Men's: Trade-Offs and Strategic Accommodations in Egyptian Women's Reproductive Lives," in Petchesky and Judd, eds., 1998.

14. Thanks to Susanna Fried for calling my attention to this point.

15. The *IPPF Charter on Sexual and Reproductive Rights* is the best example of a thorough, thoughtful compendium of basic principles (and the existing instruments from which they derive) that uses very broad language to imply—but not to specify. The closest it comes to articulating an affirmative approach to sexual pleasure is under Principle 2, "The Right to Liberty and Security of the Person," where it states, "All persons have the right to be free to enjoy and control their sexual and reproductive life, having due regard to the rights of others." Also, "All persons have the right to be free from externally imposed fear, shame, guilt, beliefs based on myths, and other psychological factors inhibiting their sexual response or impairing their sexual relationships."

References

Altman, D. (1995). "Political Sexualities: Meanings and Identities in the Time of AIDS." In Parker, R. G., and Gagnon, J. (eds.), *Conceiving Sexuality: Approaches to Sex Research in a Postmodern World*, pp. 97–106. New York and London: Routledge.

Amin, S., and Hossain, S. (1995). "Women's Reproductive Rights and the Politics of Fundamentalism: A View from Bangladesh." *American University Law Review*, 44:1319–43.

Bunch, C. (1990). "Women's Rights as Human Rights: Toward a Re-Vision of Human Rights." *Human Rights Quarterly*, 12:486–98.

Catholics for a Free Choice. (1995). *The Vatican and the Fourth World Conference on Women*. Washington, DC: Catholics for a Free Choice.

Center for Women's Global Leadership. (1996). *From Vienna to Beijing: The Global Tribunal on Accountability for Women's Human Rights*. Reilly, N. (ed.). New Brunswick, NJ: Rutgers University.

Cook, R. (1995). "Human Rights and Reproductive Self-Determination." *American University Law Review*, 44:975–1475.

Cook, R. (ed.). (1994). *Human Rights of Women: National and International Perspectives*. Philadelphia: University of Pennsylvania.

Copelon, R. (1994): "Recognizing the Egregious in the Everyday: Domestic Violence as Torture." *Columbia Human Rights Law Review*, 25:291–367.

Copelan, R., and Hernandez, B. E. (1994). *Sexual and Reproductive Rights and Health as Human Rights: Concepts and Strategies*. International Women's Human Rights Law Clinic. NY: City University of New York.

Copelan, R., and Petchesky, R. (1995). "Toward an Interdependent Approach to Reproductive and Sexual Rights as Human Rights: Reflections on the ICPD and Beyond." In Schuler, M. A. (ed.), *From Basic Needs to Basic Rights: Women's Claim to Human Rights*, 343–67. Washington, DC: Women, Law, and Development International.

Corrêa, S. (1994). *Population and Reproductive Rights: Feminist Perspectives from the South*. London: Zed Press.

Corrêa, S., and Petchesky, R. (1994). "Reproductive and Sexual Rights: A Feminist Perspective. In Germain, A., and Chen, L., (eds.), *Population Policies Reconsidered*, 107–23. Cambridge: Harvard University.

Eisenstein, Z. (1996). *Hatreds: Racialized and Sexualized Conflicts in the 21st Century*. New York and London: Routledge.

Evangelium Vitae. (1995). "Pope's Letter: A 'Sinister' World Has Led to 'Crimes Against Life.'" *New York Times*, March 31, A12–A13.

Foucault, M. (1978). *The History of Sexuality*, Vol. I, *An Introduction*. New York: Pantheon.

Freedman, L. P., and Isaacs, S. L. (1993). "Human Rights and Reproductive Choice." *Studies in Family Planning*, 24:18–30.

Heise, L. (1995). "Violence, Sexuality, and Women's Lives." In Parker, R. G., and Gagnon, J., (eds.), *Conceiving Sexuality: Approaches to Sex Research in a Postmodern World*, 109–34. New York and London: Routledge.

Human Rights Watch. (1996). *Shattered Lives: Sexual Violence during the Rwandan Genocide and Its Aftermath*. New York: Human Rights Watch.

International Planned Parenthood Federation. (1996). *IPPF Charter on Sexual and Reproductive Rights*. London: International Planned Parenthood Federation.

Leary, V. (1994). "The Right to Health in International Human Rights Law." *Health and Human Rights*, 1:24–56.

Ong, A. (1994). "State versus Islam: Malay Families, Women's Bodies, and the Body Politic in Malaysia." In *Women's Reproductive Rights in Muslim Communities and Countries: Issues and Resources*, Women Living Under Muslim Laws, Cairo, August, 26–36.

Ortiz-Ortega, A., Amuchástegui, A., and Rivas, M. (1998). " 'Because They Were Born from Me': Negotiating Women's Rights in Mexico." In Petchesky, R., and Judd, K., (eds.), *Negotiating Reproductive Rights: Women's Perspectives across Countries and Cultures*, 145–79. London and New York: Zed Press.

Osakue, G., and Martin-Hilber, A. (1998). "Women's Sexuality and Fertility in Nigeria: Breaking the Culture of Silence." In Petchesky, R., and Judd, K., (eds.), *Negotiating Reproductive Rights: Women's Perspectives across Countries and Cultures*, 180–216. London and New York: Zed Press.

Parker, R. G., and Gagnon, J. (eds.). (1995). *Conceiving Sexuality: Approaches to Sex Research in a Postmodern World*. New York and London: Routledge.

Pateman, C. (1988). *The Sexual Contract*. Stanford: Stanford University Press.

Petchesky, R. (1993). "From Population Control to Reproductive Rights: Feminist Fault Lines." *Reproductive Health Matters*, 6 (November): 152–61.

———. (1995). "The Body as Property: A Feminist Re-Vision." In Ginsburg, F., and Rapp, R., (eds.), *Conceiving the New World Order*, 387–406. Berkeley and Los Angeles: University of California Press.

———. (1997). "Spiraling Discourses of Reproductive and Sexual Rights: A Post-Beijing Assessment of International Feminist Politics." In Cohen, K., Jones, K., and Tronto, J., (eds.), *Women Question Politics*, 569–87. New York and London: Routledge.

Petchesky, R., and Judd, K. (eds.). (1998). *Negotiating Reproductive Rights: Women's Perspectives across Countries and Cultures*. London: Zed Press.

Portella, A. P., de Mello e Souza, C., and Diniz, S. (1998). "Not Like Our Mothers: Reproductive Choice and the Emergence of Citizenship among Brazilian Rural Workers, Domestic Workers, and Housewives." In Petchesky, R., and Judd, K., (eds.), *Negotiating Reproductive Rights: Women's Perspectives across Countries and Cultures*, 31–68. London and New York: Zed Press.

Romany, C. (1994). "State Responsibility Goes Private: A Feminist Critique of the Public/Private Distinction in International Human Rights Law." In Cook, R. (ed.), *Human Rights of Women: National and International Perspectives*, 85–115. Philadelphia: University of Pennsylvania.

Rosenbloom, R. (ed.). (1995). *Unspoken Rules: Sexual Orientation and Women's Human Rights*. San Francisco: International Gay and Lesbian Human Rights Commission.

Seif El Dawla, A., Hadi, A. A., and Wahab, N. A. (1997). "Women's Wit Over

Men's: Trade-Offs and Strategic Accommodations in Egyptian Women's Reproductive Lives." In Petchesky, R., and Judd, K., (eds.), *Negotiating Reproductive Rights: Women's Perspectives across Countries and Cultures*, 69–107. London and New York: Zed Press.

Sen, A. (1990). "Individual Freedom as a Social Commitment." *New York Review of Books*, June 14, 49–52/79–80.

Sen, G., and Snow, R. C. (eds.). (1994). *Power and Decision: The Social Control of Reproduction*. Cambridge: Harvard University Press.

Tambiah, Y. (1995). "Sexuality and Human Rights." In Schuler, M. A. (ed.), *From Basic Needs to Basic Rights: Women's Claim to Human Rights*, 369–90. Washington, DC: Women, Law, and Development International.

———. (1996). "Sexual Rights, the State, and Democratic Process: Issues for South Asian Women." Paper presented at the AWID Conference, Washington, DC, 5–8 September.

Toubia, N. (1995). *Female Genital Mutilation: A Call for Global Action*. New York: RAINBO. (Available from Women, Ink, 777 United Nations Plaza, New York, NY 10017.)

United Nations. (1994). *Report of the International Conference on Population and Development*. Cairo, Egypt, 5–13 September.

United Nations. (1995). *Platform for Action of the Fourth World Conference on Women*. Beijing, China, 4–15 September.

Chapter Five

Cross-National Perspectives on Gender and Power

Purnima Mane and Peter Aggleton

If we reflect for a moment on the ways HIV and AIDS have most often been conceived over the last fifteen years, one thing becomes clear. From the start, AIDS has been understood as something new— an anomaly, and a terrible one. Certainly HIV, the virus that causes the acquired immune deficiency syndrome, was new to science, and admittedly the advent of HIV disease has raised important questions about sex, sexuality, and drug use, but many issues highlighted by the epidemic, and by human responses to it, are not that new. Central among these are questions of gender and power, of sexual divisions and gender inequalities, and of how women may best be empowered in social and sexual relations with men. In this chapter, we shall examine some of these concerns in relation to recent efforts to analyze more precisely the nature of women's vulnerability to STDs and HIV, and also in relation to interventions that go beyond the teaching of 'skills' to broader concerns with power and gender relations.

There is clear evidence that women's vulnerability to HIV and AIDS is rapidly rising in both developed and developing countries; approximately 41 percent of the over thirty-three million adults living with HIV and AIDS are women; in Sub-Saharan Africa, women account for about half of all infected adults; the proportion is 35 percent in the Caribbean; in South and South East Asia around one-fourth of infections are among women, while in Latin America, around 20 percent are (UNAIDS and WHO, 1998). To state this is not to presuppose that only women are at heightened risk, nor to draw attention from other especially vulnerable social groups, such as behaviorally homosexual men, male and female sex workers, and those who share needles and syringes. It is, however, to recognize the important role that gender plays in structuring inequalities and in enhancing, for women, sexual and reproductive health risks. Support for this view is witnessed both in declarations at the International Conference on Population and Development in Cairo and the fourth World Conference on Women in Beijing, and in a growing concern to identify woman-controlled technologies that may protect against HIV infection (Elias and Heise, 1994; WHO, 1993a; Elias and Coggins, 1996).

It is against this background that we shall examine findings from a series of studies commissioned in 1992 by the World Health Organization's (then) Global Programme on AIDS, and later supported by the Joint United Nations Programme on HIV/AIDS.[1] These studies set out to examine, within the broader context of prevailing gender relations, sexual negotiation, the empowerment of women, and the female condom. Conducted by local principal investigators in Mexico (Hernandez, de Caso, and Ortiz, 1995), Costa Rica (Herrera, Elizondo, et al., 1996), Senegal (Niang, 1995), and Indonesia (Setiadi, Jatipura, and Santoso, 1995), these studies sought to examine whether the female condom could enhance women's power to negotiate for safer sex, and if so, in what circumstances and for what groups.

At the start of research, opinion was divided over the empowering potential of the female condom. It was sometimes argued this new technology held the potential to empower women by offering another way to protect themselves and their partners; on the other hand, the female condom might add further to women's responsibilities and burden with respect to sexual and reproductive health. Earlier studies, producing somewhat equivocal results with respect both to acceptability of the female condom and its empowering potential, had largely involved small and perhaps untypical samples of women (in richer countries, mainly articulate and middle-class; in the developing world, mainly sex workers). Moreover, they had not included what was likely a key variable—training and ongoing support in the use of this relatively novel form of protection.

In developing the General Research Protocol for these studies (WHO, 1993b), we had to reflect on a range of complex issues, some of which will be discussed.

First, the female condom could not easily be used surreptitiously, and so required, at the very least, acquiescence by the male partner. Thus merely making it available would not necessarily favor women's protection, in the context of imbalances in gender power. If the female condom was to serve as an empowering technology, basic issues would first need exploration. The complexity and variability of gender relations in different sociocultural settings must be better understood, and approaches to empowerment and sexual negotiation relevant to men and women in these settings would be needed. In particular, it would be necessary to remedy any deficits in women's understanding of sex and reproduction, STDs and AIDS, and to provide training in the use of the female condom and in negotiating for its use.

Second, it would be necessary to build upon the available repertoire for sexual negotiation, providing an opportunity for women to share experiences and learn new skills related to communication about sex-related protection.

Third, it would be necessary to provide social support so that such issues could be openly discussed, without fear of reprisal and recrimination, by groups of women, and finally, it would be necessary to better understand how economic and social factors impinged upon and affected women's ability and opportunity to use the information and understanding they acquired.

The Studies

Concern with these issues led to design of a two-part study to be conducted in the four sites mentioned above. The first part took the form of an in-depth ethnographic study of gender relations, particularly in the area of sex. Using close-focus techniques, efforts were made, in each site, to explore the prevailing climate of gender relations, both in partnerships not involving direct exchange of money or goods for sex, and in situations of sex work. Data was collected through in-depth interviews, focus group discussions, and direct observation of the settings for sex-related social exchanges between women and men. Both women and men were interviewed to elicit contrasting as well as shared perspectives on the normative patterns and the lived realities of gender relations.

The second part of the study involved in-depth analysis of responses, by women and by their partners, to the female condom after it was introduced, in each site, through controlled intervention. Two contrasting groups of women were involved at this stage, those actively involved in sex work at the time and those not, to explore any differences in response within, and between, groups. The female condom itself was introduced only after a series of participatory educational sessions providing information on sex, sexuality, reproduction, STDs, and AIDS. These sessions allowed individual and group reflection on feelings and attitudes about sexual relationships, as well as consideration of current patterns of sexual negotiation. Subsequent to these introductory sessions and distribution of the female condoms, interim sessions were arranged for women to discuss initial experiences with this condom and any problems occurring through its use. Possible solutions were identified, and group support provided. The General Research Protocol aimed to provide not merely a new protective device but also collectively empowering experiences whereby women could acquire the confidence, skills, and support necessary to negotiate its use. Thus the study went well beyond previous inquiries into the female condom's acceptability, in recognizing that acceptability may be determined as much by how the technology is introduced as by its physical characteristics.

The local investigations were carried out, except in Senegal, primarily in urban areas and involved women of varying socioeconomic status. Each of the two groups of women involved at each site numbered twenty to thirty. The studies should therefore be seen as preliminary explorations of what can be achieved, in both sex-work and non-sex-work contexts, when the female condom is introduced along with training and support in its use.

Prevailing Gender Relations

To better understand women's responses and reactions to the female condom, it was necessary to understand aspects of prevailing gender relations in the four contexts studied. In each, gender relations may best be characterized by overall inequality. In Costa Rica, Mexico, and Indonesia, for example, women were expected to take the main responsibility for domestic and caring tasks within their household regardless of whether they also engaged in paid outside employment. Often the women had a resignation or fatalism about this situation. As one women in Mexico put it, "According to what we have been taught, women should take care of the home, children, and husband. We weren't taught to see ourselves as equal to men." Normatively also, they were expected to submit to their husbands' requests for sex, as and when these occurred. As one women in Indonesia stated, "I don't feel right to refuse because it's sinful. A woman is her husband's property, she is already bought. It is appropriate to have sex once or twice a week." A similar sentiment was expressed by a respondent in Senegal, "A sane mind cannot imagine how a spouse could refuse to have sexual intercourse with her husband."

We should be careful not to see in these remarks a passivity or weakness that was not there. Many women expressed concern about what they perceived as their position, and economic changes were having an impact on the division of labor within and outside the household. In Mexico, where women comprise thirty-three percent of the economically active workforce, a minority of "liberated" women was visible in the study—women making strenuous efforts to live their relationships with men differently than before, often as lovers rather than wives, in conscious efforts to shake off centuries of oppression. As one such women said, "A clandestine relationship is more enjoyable, going out with a man who is committed [married or with a regular girlfriend or partner] is better than with someone who is there only for me, and who, because of that, begins to limit my freedom." Among the non-sex-worker groups studied in Senegal, where men are permitted under Moslem law to have as many as four wives, a particularly strict gendered division of labor pertained. Men were expected to provide the home and foodstuff for the household; women were responsible for the production of foodstuffs for ceremonies, and for gift-giving and hospitality. But even here, in the context of increasing economic crisis, changes were taking place with women increasingly taking over, at the household level, in times of need, what had previously been seen as men's responsibilities and areas of work.

Women sex workers participating in the studies also were, in each site, influenced by prevailing patterns of gender relations. The majority had spouses or regular partners, as well as paying clients or men who gave gifts and other favors in exchange for sex. In the former "primary" relationships, much the same division of labor pertained as with women not involved in sex work. Additionally, whereas sex with clients was most usually seen as routine or mechanical, sex with regular partners or spouses was seen as more emotionally fulfilling. One woman in Costa Rica said, when describing her regular partner, "I like that he treats me well, makes me feel like a woman. He's not being charged for the service, and one really feels it. The clients make me feel like a robot."

Clearly, we should in all contexts guard against too static an analysis of gender relations, and in every setting be open to the ways women may challenge men's power in social and sexual relationships. Nowhere was this conclusion more clear than regarding the complexity of communication about sex and reproductive relationships.

Communication and "Negotiation" about Sex

While, in each setting, dominant beliefs and expectations suggested that women lacked power in relationships with men, rendering "negotiation" about sexual (or other) matters highly problematic, in practice things were not so clearcut. In spite of overall subordination to men, women were far from powerless in their everyday lives, able to use a range of strategies to influence social and sexual relationships with men.

While sexual matters and sexual needs could not often be discussed openly—as one woman in Costa Rica put it "[I cannot talk about what *I* want] because a man would get upset if I said it to him so directly" such matters could be communicated in less obtrusive ways, either nonverbally or by using local cultural resources. In Senegal, for example, erotic clothing and perfumes were used by women to communicate readiness and availability for sex—in ways enabling significant control over the sexual domain. Thus, while husbands might possess conjugal rights to intercourse, they did not possess the same rights to erotic services as to domestic services, since erotic services were viewed as gifts that a woman could withdraw if her needs were not also met. As one woman stated, "Before such generosity can be shown by the use of erotic products and practices, men are under the obligation to satisfy the woman's desires; otherwise the man is demeaned in the eyes of the woman and no longer seen to merit such generosity." In Indonesia, casual touch, a provocative and unusual display of a body part normally concealed, or reference to the husband's "duty" were common strategies to initiate sex. In Costa Rica and Mexico, postures, gestures, and displays of affection were used to signal desire and sexual readiness.

A comparable range of strategies existed to indicate unavailability or a reluctance to engage in specific sexual acts. In Indonesia, for example, women could influence the nature of sexual practices and acts by recourse to cultural and religious taboos prohibiting, for example, oral sex: "A mouth is the place for eating, talking, not for doing sexual intercourse." In Costa Rica, some women reported using such subversive techniques to avoid sex as avoiding physical contact with their regular male partners, feigning exhaustion or illness, or expressing a need to sleep. In Senegal, local rules determined when sex could be refused by a woman—for example, in the daytime, during menses, while breast feeding, and on nights reserved for the co-wife in a polygynous marriage. Additionally, in Senegal local beliefs about sexual probity helped women in their "negotiations" with men. It was believed, for example, that any child born as a result of forced sex would be deficient in some way.[2]

Levels of verbal communication about the nature and context of sex were higher among sex workers and their clients than among women and their husbands or regular partners, but even here there were limits to what could be discussed. In all sites, responsibility for negotiating safer sex rested largely with the individual woman, who, besides seeking to negotiate condom use, might try to impose limits on the sexual acts permissible (e.g., typically no anal sex in Mexico, no oral or anal sex in Indonesia). A range of techniques might be used to persuade a man that condom use was desirable—flattery, statements of its value for *both* parties, pointing out that it offered protection against pregnancy, and, on rare occasions, threats of STDs and HIV.

The social and legal context, including the "rules" set by sex-work venue managers, also influenced negotiation. In Costa Rica and Mexico, and in contexts where condom use was relatively normative, women needed less time and effort to persuade clients to use condoms. In Senegal, there were important differences between registered and non-registered sex workers in negotiating for safer sex. Whereas the former had a relatively high degree of influence over acts engaged in, price charged, and context in which sex took place, the latter, not wishing to be publicly seen as prostitutes, were more dependent upon their male partners when negotiating form and content of the sexual encounter.

It is important not to draw too stark a distinction between the form of sexual negotiation in sex-work and non-sex-work contexts. In many married relationships, for example, a woman looked upon sex not so much as a right of the male partner but as an exchangeable commodity—to be used to obtain affection, to secure harmonious relationships at home, to achieve social status, and to obtain favors, benefits, and goods, both for herself and for her children. On the whole, however, such negotiating potential was kept "secret" by women who saw this as a hidden power—although one recognized in the abstract by both sexes and which could be used, within limits, to women's benefit. In Mexico, for example, women's capacity to use this potential depended upon their socioeconomic situation, their desire to maintain status, their access to new ideas and ideologies, their degree of security in the relationship, the presence or absence of children to "negotiate," emotional dependence on the relationship, fear of loneliness, and other variables.

The previous discussion should make clear that women's ability to "negotiate" over sexual matters is both enabled and constrained by context-specific cultural and situational variables. These, and the more pervasive gender relations that frame them, offer a context in which to make sense of responses to a new protective technology such as the female condom. Without an understanding of these factors, and how they both *enable* and *constrain* women in sexual negotiations with men, it is impossible either to predict or to understand responses to the female condom in any particular setting. But other factors, too, influence how the female condom is taken up and used. Central among these are influences relating to how the female condom is introduced to women and their sexual partners.

Responses to the Female Condom

It is important first to say something about responses to other barrier methods of protection, in particular the male condom, at each site, in order to establish a context against which to view responses to the female condom itself.

Condom use in marriage or in regular non-sex-work partnerships was reportedly low in all sites where the study took place, not only because of negative associations but also because of the high value placed on fertility (in some sites), of religious taboos against condom use, of poor condom quality locally, and of low confidence levels, among men using the condom, about its use. Additionally, in Senegal women reported that, for their male partners, sex was not complete without ejaculation into the vagina, and it was widely believed by women that men pierced holes in the end of the condom to allow such successful completion of the sexual act. In Indonesia, condom use was reported virtually nonexistent outside sex-work contexts.

In all four sites, male condom use was reported as more common within the context of sex work. When it came to negotiating male condom use, sex workers in all sites reported employing persuasion, flattery, appeal to customers' sense of well-being, and other techniques. These were skills used more generally in sex work to "negotiate" price, kind of sex to take place, where sex would occur, and so on. As we had suspected, many women sex workers reported being relatively skilled in communicating to men what they would and would not do, although economic need, force of circumstance, and the refusal of men to cooperate meant that, on occasion, women were forced to practice unsafe sex when they desired not to.

As for women's experience using the female condom, responses were extremely positive. In contrast to their initial expectations—that the condom would be too large or small, be too uncomfortable or slip out—women in both sex-work and non-sex-work contexts reported enhanced pleasure and security, and feeling of more control of the sexual act. In almost every case where the woman was able to "negotiate" the use of the condom with her male partner, initial anxieties were lessened. Where negative feelings persisted, they tended to be linked to discomfort caused to the man by the internal ring, and/or discomfort to the woman from the external ring. A minority of respondents reported finding the female condom too noisy or too slippery.

In Costa Rica, women talked openly about the enhanced power the female condom gave, one saying, "It is like having control, power. Apart from that, it feels good." In Mexico, a woman commented, "It feels really great. You feel really free. Oh it's the best invention since birth control, and I like it even better than the male condom because . . . you can control the situation. You are taking care of yourself, and you don't depend on another person." In Senegal, women reported that their male partners experienced enhanced sexual pleasure with the female condom, which in some cases became incorporated in activities undertaken as prelude to intercourse. As one woman said, "When my husband wanted to have sexual intercourse with me, be it at night or early in the morning, he went to look for the woman's condom himself, tore open the sachet, and placed it in my vagina with gestures which pleased me as much as they did him." The negative views expressed tended to come from women whose knowledge of their own anatomy was limited, or who felt sex was something unpleasant or dirty.

Among sex workers, the female condom provided additional leverage in the "negotiation" process with clients. In Mexico, some women were able to charge more for sex when their client did not wear a male condom, or Indonesia, where the female condom was a means to bargain with clients over protection: "With a 'friend,' it is up to him. With a customer I don't know, I will insist on using a condom. If not a male condom, then I will offer the female condom, or no transaction." In Senegal, some sex workers reported that the additional lubrication offered by the female condom made their clients ejaculate faster—"Now, with the female condom's lubrication, my partners ejaculate rapidly, which tires me less—and besides, in place of pain, I feel more smoothness."

What factors were responsible for the responses we have documented, and what leads do they offer on promoting the uptake of a new protective and potentially empowering technology in other contexts? Clearly, from an exploratory study such as this, it is difficult to identify with certainty the key factors determining successful uptake and use. Nevertheless, some insight can be gained from the women's responses. Nearly all reports suggest that the crucial factor was the women's active participation in the intervention element of the study. Most respondents, for example, reported that the most critical change was not in sexual relations but in *themselves*. In Indonesia, for example, women reported having gained new experiences and understandings from participation in the workshops and other activities. As a result, they had felt more able to communicate with their partners about protection and about STDs and AIDS in a culturally appropriate manner. In Mexico, one woman was reported saying, "After the workshops, it's like you find more words to talk to them differently, and they feel good with the condom. That was when the change happened and I decided I have a voice and a vote, and it is not only his decision. I have a right to feel loved and desired."

Looking closely at the methodologies of the studies described, in comparison with those reporting difficulties in acceptance, one thing becomes plain. A prerequisite for success appears to be the education, training, and support that accompanied the introduction of the condom, and that continued throughout the study as women shared their experiences and their partners' reactions. Typically activities took the form of initial group discussions about gender relations, sex, and communication with partners, followed by instruction in how to use the female condom, practice in its use, interview of women after they tried the condom, and collective reflection on the experience. Earlier studies, including the majority of investigations conducted in Europe and North America, marginalized consideration of prevailing gender relations, of patterns of communication about sexual matters, and of situations and contexts for introduction of the female condom. Instead, the female condom was, typically, simply made available, as if all that was required for its successful use was availability and an individual's desire to try it.

Of course, much of this is not new. In a recent paper for the Joint United Nations Programme on HIV/AIDS (UNAIDS), Geeta Rao Gupta (1995) identifies the following factors among those influencing gender power as it operates in and around HIV prevention : (1) access to information; (2) access to skills and economic resources; (3) access to appropriate services and technologies; and (4) access to social support, including supportive social norms. Many of these influences were explicitly addressed by the studies reported here. In accordance with the specifications of the General Research Protocol, efforts were made to make good any deficits in women's understanding of sex, of reproductive anatomy and physiology, of STDs and AIDS, of women's vulnerability to these infections, and so on. Steps were also taken, through participatory learning, to provide opportunities for women to share and develop skills related to communication about protection. Principal investigators and their teams at each site tried hard to nurture social support among peers so as to offer a supportive environment for learning and reflection. Of course, women were provided the resources whereby to protect themselves and their partners from sex-related risks. The above process encouraged women to introduce the female condom in ways most appropriate to themselves, both individually and culturally, and this we feel is a prerequisite for the effectiveness of any future intervention that seeks to empower women in their "negotiations" (sexual or other) with men. Clearly, more extended evaluation will be needed to confirm or deny the validity of these claims. But we should perhaps be encouraged by these preliminary findings—not least because they suggest there may be ways of working with women and their communities that can show real benefit both for the women and for their sexual partners.

Perhaps as important, the studies suggest new ways of thinking about women's sexual empowerment in relation to their sexual and reproductive health. In particular, the studies highlight the importance of adopting a culturally specific, situated, multi-dimensional perspective—one that views empowerment as a continuum rather than as a final product. What empowerment in sexual negotiation means to the women in Indonesia who participated in this study clearly differs, in many respects, from what it means to those in Mexico, and both differ from what it means to those in Senegal. And within each context, there exist structured differences between those women involved in sex work and those not.[3] Although, on the whole, the former had relative autonomy over the form and context within which sexual relations occurred (at least with clients), the latter were more constrained. These are important points, raising important questions about the universality (or restrictedness) of concepts like empowerment, and thus encouraging respect for the diversity of ways women and men may seek to communicate over sexual and reproductive matters, and the multiple opportunities for "negotiation" that such communication allows.

Acknowledgments

We would like to acknowledge the work of the principal investigators of the studies referred to in this chapter: Gisela Herrera and Jorge Elizondo in Costa Rica, Bernadette Setiadi in Indonesia, Griselda Hernandez in Mexico, and Cheikh Niang in Senegal. With their teams, they provided much of the data from which the analysis presented here has been developed. We would also like to thank Sue Scott, from the University of Stirling, in the United Kingdom, who worked with us on the comparative analysis of findings from the studies.

Notes

1. The findings, interpretations, and views expressed in this paper are entirely those of the authors, and do not necessarily reflect official policy or positions of the Joint United Nations Programme on HIV/AIDS (UNAIDS).
2. There are contradictions here since, within the same communities,

although acceptable for neighbors to intervene were a man to beat a woman during the daytime, it would be less so for them to do so at night, when it would be assumed that the cause of the beating was a refusal to have sex.

3. It is important to recognise that the majority of women sex workers in this study were not formally "bonded" to their work in ways possibly characterizing sex work contexts where children and young people may be sold into prostitution by their parents, or where an "indentured" system of labour exists.

References

Elias, C. J., and Coggins, C. (1996). "Female-Controlled Methods to Prevent Sexual Transmission of HIV." *AIDS*, 10(suppl 3):S43–S51.

Elias, C. J., and Heise, L. (1994). *The Development of Microbicides: A New Method of HIV Prevention for Women*. The Population Council, Programme Division, Working Papers, no. 6. New York: Population Council.

Hernandez, G., de Caso, L. E., and Ortiz, V. O. (1995). *Sexual Negotiation, Female Empowerment, and the Female Condom in Mexico*. Final report to UNAIDS. Unpublished.

Herrera, G., Elizondo, J., et al. (1996). *Negociación Sexual, Empoderamiento de las Mujeres, y Condón Femenino*. Ministerio de Salud, Republica de Costa Rica. Final report to UNAIDS. Unpublished.

Niang, C. I. (1995). *Sexual Negotiations and the Use of Women's Condom in Kolda and Kaolack, Senegal*. Final report to UNAIDS. Unpublished.

Rao Gupta, G. (1995). *Integrating a Gender Perspective in UNAIDS Policies and Programs—A Proposed Strategy*. Unpublished.

Setiadi, B. N., Jatipura, I., and Santoso, G. (1995). *Sexual Negotiation, the Empowerment of Women, and the Female Condom*. Final report to UNAIDS. Unpublished.

UNAIDS and World Health Organization. (1998). *AIDS Epidemic Update: 1998* (December). Geneva.

World Health Organization. (1993a). *Report of a Meeting on the Development of Vaginal Microbicides for the Prevention of Heterosexual Transmission of HIV*. Global Programme on AIDS, Geneva, 11–13 November.

———. (1993b). *General Research Protocol for Studies of Sexual Negotiation, the Empowerment of Women, and the Female Condom*. Social and Behavioural Studies and Support Unit, Global Programme on AIDS, Geneva.

Chapter Six

Gender Stereotypes and Power Relations

Unacknowledged Risks for STDs in Argentina

Mónica Gogna and Silvina Ramos

There is a growing consensus on the insensitivity of most STD/HIV-related health education and promotion programs to the psychosocial and cultural dimensions of health–illness behavior (Cleary, 1988; Parker, 1992; Campbell, 1995). The international scientific community is gradually accepting that, for an educational intervention to be effective in changing behavior, it should be based upon an understanding of how a group of people perceives, conceptualizes, and finds meaning in its social and physical worlds. Consensus is also growing on the need to take into account social and cultural norms and expectations regarding interlocking cultural domains, such as sexuality and gender (WHO, 1993; de Zalduondo and Bernard, 1995; Dixon-Mueller, 1993; Rao Gupta and Weiss, 1995).

This chapter deals with the cultural and psychosocial dimensions of STDs, a particularly neglected area of research that has recently become a focus of concern, as a result of the HIV/AIDS epidemic. The report covers results of a study conducted in Buenos Aires, Argentina, aimed at fostering understanding of preventive and treatment behavior vis-à-vis STDs. The study used qualitative data collection techniques—focus-groups and in-depth interviews—and two systematic data collection techniques (free list and pile sort). The population studied consisted of low-income youth and adults, both male and female, sampled from a neighborhood in Greater Buenos Aires.[1] The interviews and group sessions were taped, and data were analyzed using qualitative data management programs.

We show existing links between three cultural domains: health/illness, sexuality, and gender. We also seek to unveil the multilayer, dynamic nature of these domains, and the fact that prescriptions emanating from each may reinforce or neutralize one another. More specifically, we develop two basic ideas. First, lay beliefs regarding STDs are strongly tinted by deeply rooted ideas regarding gender identities, gender relations, and sexual matters. Second, STDs have a very special social and cultural meaning that greatly affects prevention and treatment behavior.

We further raise some implications of our research findings for the design of culturally appropriate educational strategies to encourage individuals to adopt preventive and treatment behaviors. To succeed, such strategies need to be especially sensitive to the trade-offs people face when making "health decisions" affecting sexual life; their choices usually involve undoubtedly complex issues like trust, love, pleasure, and self-esteem.

Given this complexity, our theoretical approach took elements from several sources: the health belief model (Hochbaum, 1981; Rosenstock, 1960, 1966; Rosenstock and Becker, 1974; Rosenstock and Kirscht, 1974; Suchman, 1965; Mechanic, 1978; Becker and Maiman, 1983); lay notions of health and illness (Freidson, 1978; Fitzpatrick, 1984); feminist theory (Giele, 1988; Benería and Roldán, 1992; Rubin, 1992); and the social constructivist approach to sexuality (Giddens, 1992; Gagnon, 1988 and 1990 [on "scripting theory"]; Laumann et al., 1994).

STD prevention and treatment are considered health-seeking behaviors influenced by classic determinants of individual behavior regarding health and illness. Among the most important are perceived susceptibility, perceived severity of the consequences of the disease, perceived costs of preventive and treatment measures, availability and quality of information on the disease, and evaluation of the efficacy of available treatments.

Nonetheless, since STDs involve sexuality, it is likely the classic health belief model is insufficient. Sexuality is a facet of human behavior generally engulfed in prohibitions, taboos, and preconceptions that prevent open discussion of disease-related issues involving the genitals and thus affect recognition, prevention, and treatment of STDs. The adoption of preventive and treatment behavior entails introducing an element of rationality into a realm of human existence that is emotionally loaded, and eventually a certain interference in the very intimate aspects of a person's life that are seldom open to others. And since the sexual bond implies a relation between two persons, the prevention and treatment of STDs is subject to the dynamic of the attachment and must inevitably involve, by action or omission, both participants.

In addition, the gender dimension cuts straight through STDs; these diseases affect men and women in biologically and culturally different ways. "It is not only more likely that a noninfected woman will acquire STDs from an infected partner than vice versa, but it is also more probable that she will suffer more serious consequences in the long run, such as inflammatory pelvic disease, ectopic pregnancy, cancer of the cervix, chronic pelvic pain, or infertility" (Dixon-Mueller and Wasserheit, 1991). Also, STDs are more frequently asymptomatic in women than in men. To this "biological sexism" we should add cultural sexism, since women are often blamed for the spread of STDs (McCormack, 1982). And gender stereotypes and the double sexual moral standard (which differentially sanctions the exercise of sexuality by men and women) have a bearing on the ability of men and women to adopt appropriate self-care behavior.

Finally, although STD prevention and treatment are matters of health-care behavior, they really imply changes in sexual behavior. Thus a comprehensive approach to the health problem requires understanding this particular "form of conduct, intricately related to pleasure, sin, reproduction, aging, growth, and loss—among other things—that is sexuality" (Gagnon, 1990).

How the Ethnomedical Model of STDs Affects Health-Seeking Behavior

A striking quality of lay concepts of health and illness is their complexity. Lay ideas are seldom formalized or integrated, and frequently are expressed tentatively and hesitantly.[2] They are also syncretic in origin—that is, they are derived from a variety of sources and respond to experience in a flexible manner and according to an individual's current concerns. Further, lay concepts not only involve an alternative set of entities and causes than those of medicine, but act as condensed symbols that refer to a wider variety of cultural experiences. As Fitzpatrick indicates, "Lay concepts of illness do not merely name entities in the body but are powerful images associated with other realms of life" (Fitzpatrick et al., 1984, 21).

In this section we describe and analyze the composition of the "ethnomedical model of STDs," and try to show how lay beliefs about causes, symptoms, forms of transmission, consequences, and the sociocultural meaning of these illnesses affect perceived severity, thus affecting health-seeking behavior. We also highlight gender concordances and differences regarding these matters.

The central concern of the study was to understand how people conceive of STDs and whether they relate STDs to sexual life in any way. Given these interests, an emic perspective was emphasized,[3] and the initial question, in both focus groups and in-depth interviews, was "What are the health problems people may have that relate to their sexual life?"[4]

The study population identified a wide and heterogeneous range of terms. The list included only three medical terms (syphilis, AIDS, and HPV) but included: some terms from common language (*purgación* ["purging"], *pudrición* ["rotting" and "fungus"]); other terms referring to a generic affliction ("infections"); others designating fluids ("discharge," "women's internal problems," "strong menstruation," for example), or specific problems appearing in the "nether area" (for example, "hemorrhoids," "urinary infections"); and the old and well-known expression for STDs, "venereal diseases."[5]

It is interesting that men and women did not recall identical sets of "health problems related to sexual life." Men reported almost twice as many terms as did women (twenty-one and twelve, respectively), and only seven terms were named by both men and women ("venereal diseases," "flux," "fungus," "urinary infection," "crab lice," "syphilis," and "AIDS"). Both sexes referred most to AIDS. With this exception, the more frequently mentioned diseases by men and women differ. Among men, "rotting,"[6] crab lice, and fungus, were the problems most cited. Women mentioned syphilis, vaginal infections, "venereal diseases," and fungus. The terms—and the problems—seemed to be gender-oriented. Men not only recognized a wider spectrum of problems but listed both male and female problems. They also exhibited a wider vocabulary to describe STDs, using different words for the same problem. In contrast, women had a narrower list of terms, and the majority could be cataloged as women's problems (vaginal infections, sores, warts, flux)—the exception being AIDS, syphilis, and "venereal diseases."

This gender difference in terms used was also evidenced in regard to willingness to discuss these issues socially. The men were more determined and explicit than the women in discussing these themes with peers, frequently resorting to jokes, scoffing, or coarse expression.[7] The men's ease seems to indicate greater familiarity with this topic of conversation, due to personal experience and gender socialization. In contrast, the women proved more reluctant[8]; they found it difficult to anchor the conversation and frequently shifted to other topics (such as, the partner/relationship, infidelity, or contraception).

The lay models of causality included very different types of transmission and roots for the different diseases. In the case of AIDS, models varied from the unspecified and uncontrollable—"AIDS is everywhere," "AIDS can be transmitted in many ways"—to more precise transmission processes, such as sexual contact and blood transmission through injectable drugs, wounds or cuts, and transfusions. In relation to sexual contact, there was evident confusion about the specific mechanism producing contagion: "I don't know what it's about, maybe the blood gets it altogether in there [the vagina]" (male, age 28).

Although sexual transmission was recognized as the main source of HIV/AIDS contagion, the interviewees described only blood transmission situations—"if you get stuck with the needle of someone who has AIDS," "if a drop of blood falls on you." A greater ability to conceptualize blood transmission than sexual transmission was also reported by Loyola (1994). That study associated this evidence with the fact that, in the local health culture studied, blood was a central element in explaining organic functioning and the health–illness process. We can speculate that the population in our study found it difficult to imagine that seminal fluid could transmit disease, as this fluid is locally deemed a symbol of vitality—which cannot be associated with anything that damages or spoils. This idea of semen as a "noble fluid" contrasts with the widely extended "common sense" notion of menstruation and "strong flux" as vehicles of STDs—and as dangerous fluids with special pollution powers that weaken men, a belief prevalent, in the sample, among almost all men but few women.[9]

Particularly recognized as a source of transmission was sexual contact including "casual sexual encounters"—a term meaning very frequent sexual contact, occasional sexual encounters, and/or sexual encounters with a stranger. These forms of sexual meetings were thought to inevitably imply "erroneous selection" of the sexual partner, thus further endangering the participants—a belief reinforced by another that considers "knowing the person" an efficacious and operative defense: "Know who you are with. Surround yourself with people you can trust" (female, age 27).

The idea that STDs are transmitted by women had broad consensus among the male population studied, and some interviewees went so far as to suggest that STDs originated in women. As might be expected from the wider literature, women were often blamed for the spread of STDs.[10] Some of the men related STDs to some particular category of women ("women of the street," "women of the night," "dirty women"), but the majority mentioned that friends or acquaintances had contracted STDs from "women." Popular expressions transmitted the idea that women "rot" men ("a woman rotted him"), "do them wrong," or pass on STDs to them.

The heavy menstruation that women have is what makes all these diseases, that's what they have . . . (Male, age 42, married)

I know people who have been sick because they had sex with a woman. (Male, age 46, divorced)

He had sex only with her and she was the one who rotted him. I don't know if it's because he was weak or she was very strong. Because she was a girl of the streets. I don't know. He was always rotting. (Male, age 35, married)

It is worth highlighting that some women also blamed women, indicating that one of the most important causes and forms of STD transmission is "being with different women" ("different" in this case meaning multiple women who, also, were not like the respondent). Attributing the transmission of STDs to women was, however, generally a male argument.

Another declared cause of STDs was bodily weakness owing to depression, poor nutrition, hard work, or low defenses. This idea was stressed by men, and derived from belief that strong flux might carry "bad things" particularly risky if a man is not healthy. This idea was clearly expressed in the following: "Rotting is when you're sleeping with someone. The girl has this strong discharge and you're weak and you rot. From the strong discharge she has" (male, aged 20).

Finally, special attention was given to lack of personal care and unclean surroundings as vehicles of STD transmission.[11] Ascribing the absence of hygienic habits as causes, men were particularly concerned that some persons did not wash their genitals after sexual intercourse. The hygiene problem was sometimes associated with promiscuous practices: "They don't wash and they do it over and over and over again. The time comes when the girl rots. When you do it with her, you get it" (male, age 28).

In speaking about the "environmental route" of STDs, men and women alike described infection through unclean linen, exchange of underwear, and dirty bathrooms. It is probably because, as is well known, men are more frequent users of public bathrooms than women that these men devoted a long time to discussing the possibility of acquiring an STD through this source.[12]

To sum up, the population we studied could not attribute STDs to only one cause. Men and women alike indicated a wide range of sources, such as lack of personal hygiene, "naturally strong flux," poor selection of sexual partners, and unclean surroundings. This multiplicity of origins, requiring different preventive strategies, may explain this population's difficulties in taking effective precautions. The severity of STDs was expressed in terms of symptoms and consequences. The symptoms reported were diverse and varied widely between men and women, in terms both of specificity and of the magnitude of alarm expressed.

Only AIDS, in our population's discussions, was seen as displaying a shared set of specific and unmistakable symptoms: blemishes, hair loss, and acute thinness. At the same time, references to differences between the infected and the ill were full of confusions and inaccuracies: carriers are easier to identify; carriers do not transmit the virus; there are both healthy and unhealthy carriers; either only the man or only the woman can infect while a carrier; ill persons infect less than do carriers, since weaker. It would seem that the notion of a "healthy carrier"—that is, someone who neither looks nor feels ill and yet has and can transmit the virus—is difficult to conceptualize.[13] These confusions, and the pre-eminence of symptoms characterizing the terminal phase of the illness in our interviewees' discourse, may explain the scant predisposition of the population to adopt "safer" sexual behavior. More concretely, the emphasis on the idea that "knowing the person" is the best prevention against AIDS seems to fit with the idea that someone with AIDS can be easily identified.

The symptoms associated with other STDs differed between men and women. The former were very precise and assertive in identifying a group of "male symptoms," and highlighted the fact that these were unmistakable—burning, pain, suppuration, swelling, itching, physical weakness, and the inability to penetrate. The intensity of discomfort and pain that characterize male symptoms explains why men are so prompt to seek treatment. Men also recognized a distinct sign in a woman, namely, the unpleasant odor of "bad flux," "You can smell it half a block away." Although acknowledging this unquestionable evidence, they also showed deep concern about being unable to recognize that a woman is carrying this kind of disease, given the hiddenness—mysterious and threatening—of women's genitals: "What happens is that in a man you can see what he has, but you can't tell what a girl has inside; outside she looks fine, everything is all right, and inside she's real rotten. You don't know what she's got inside; she's got a disease you can get but you can't see it; you realize after you slept with her and you got caught . . . you can't tell what a woman has unless she tells you" (male, age 32, married).

Women's reference to symptoms were vaguer than men's. Colored flux and strong smelling flux were most often cited. However, women's discourse showed that flux was also associated with vital but undisturbing situations, such as the beginning of sexual life, the insertion of an IUD, or menopause. For women, then, the most explicit evidence was perceived both as an indication of a problem and as a part of ordinary physiological processes. Such a perception of signs as conventional and not so critical did not encourage the adoption of health-seeking behavior. Further, that these diseases are more frequently asymptomatic in women formed yet another obstacle.

Another difficulty was that symptoms could exist and be felt in one partner but not be noticeable in the other. For some, this situation was very difficult to understand; they knew that STDs are transmitted from one person to another, and were puzzled that only one had symptoms. This situation reinforced reactions of distrust or suspicion.

Regarding the consequences of STDs, both men and women stressed the emotional and conjugal problems that might arise between a couple if an STD appeared. The breakdown of the marriage, violent reactions, the sense "it will never be the same," and the destruction of the family were only some of the catastrophic consequences imagined. Moreover, their emphasis on the interpersonal conflicts that might appear (latently or manifestly) with disclosure of an STD, suggested they thought it better not to risk asking or talking about such sensitive problems. Only a few persons considered there was need for dialogue, mutual understanding, and compassion.[14]

While sharing these concerns about the emotional effects of STDs, men and women contrasted in perception of the severity of physical consequences. Manifestly feared by men, a variety of fantasies, with all their symbolic connotation, surfaced about loss of the penis as a consequence of extreme disregard to symptoms ("a little more and they have to cut it off," "it's so rotten that it falls to pieces"). Another negative consequence feared by men was the disruptive effect of STDs on sexual life. For women, in contrast, it seemed as if there were no negative physical outcomes at all; *only one* remarked about the eventual negative impact of STDs on women's future fertility, and none made reference to any impact of STDs on a woman's sexual life. Physical consequences, then, appeared much more negative and concrete for men than for women. Although women did express some unspecified concern about the consequences of STDs in terms of "men bringing the plague home," it is our hypothesis that this expression refers more to the symbolic value of STDs as diseases that "break up the family."

The perceived costs and evaluation of different preventive and treatment measures showed concordances and discrepancies between men and women. For both genders, avoiding STDs was clearly evaluated as possible, and implied the same strategy, use of male condom.[15] But implementation of this strategy was differently conceived. For women, it was a matter of the partner using condoms in secondary relationships. For men, it presupposed condom use only with select women, easy to detect as potential STD carriers: "If I haven't got a condom, I do it anyway. Depending on who the woman is. Some women are half crazy. But you can tell. From how they act, how they dress. Some women have tattoos on their arms. Then you really have to think about sleeping with her. I don't take risks often, not all of the time" (male, age 21, married).

Men and women were confident they could select partners who did not put them at risk. But this strategy worked differently for each gender. For men, it was a question of distinguishing between a housewife and another type of woman (for example, a woman of the streets, a "crazy," a woman with a very active sexual life). The first was dependable and the condom unnecessary, whereas one had to take care with the second. Women, in contrast, made their selection by "knowing the person well"—that is, knowing what he was like, where he lived, what he did, what his family was like, whom he had gone out with. These references and conditions made it possible to build up the necessary trust and, with it, self-protection.

Finally, men and women spoke about another strategy, one that implied a reciprocal fidelity: "Have a safe woman, that's yours and nobody else's, and don't wander around," although women expressed some doubts about the viability of this solution considering the "natural infidelity drive" of men.

Treatment options were also differently perceived. For men, they seemed efficacious and simple to implement. For women, treatment always implied problems, including emotional problems related to the need for the partner's compliance and practical problems regarding the use of ovules—additionally perceived as of low efficacy:

I know that with a couple of injections of antibiotics everything goes away. It's easy. I don't worry about it. (Male, age 32, separated)

This business with the ovules is a big complication, first they're difficult to put in and after, sooner or later, you get it again. (Female, age 27, married)

Finally, we would like to highlight the symbolic connotations of these diseases. In the local culture, STDs are charged with negative values and connotations because they are associated with promiscuity and lack of personal care. For men—and, to a lesser extent, women—they are diseases propagated through women. Given this cultural context, STDs have an element of shame and humiliation for a woman, since they make her appear unclean or promiscuous. Fears of social, emotional, and conjugal consequences often take priority over fears of health consequences, making women reluctant to inform male partners of symptoms or to inquire about the partner's health status or sexual behavior. For some women, the eventual risk of being beaten or abandoned, or of losing a source of emotional or financial support, far exceeds the perceived health risk of an STD. As already pointed out in the literature, "In many cultures, women accept vaginal discharges, discomfort during intercourse, or even the chronic abdominal pain which accompanies some STDs as an inevitable part of their womanhood" (Dixon-Mueller and Wasserheit, 1991, 11).

For the population studied, the set of health problems identified with sexual life did not constitute a group of diseases either serious or clearly defined in terms of symptoms, causes, or forms of transmission. This finding does not strictly apply to AIDS, which seemed more appropriately conceptualized, although some misconceptions and lack of information were observed. Data also showed that men and women had significantly different views, experiences, awareness, and information about STDs. The negative symbolic value and perceived emotional consequences of these illnesses explain the lack of awareness and concern about them, and help make understandable the barriers people (particularly women) would face on having to acknowledge an infection (thereby classifying themselves as careless, dirty, or promiscuous) and/or to seek consultation about treatment.

These lay notions about STDs and their cultural significance do not operate in isolation. They are linked to—and, in some way, reinforced by—cultural norms and prescriptions about what is expected of men and of women regarding sexual life and gender behaviors.

How Do Cultural Norms of Sexuality and Gender Stereotypes Affect Prevention and Treatment?

STDs are diseases that involve sexuality. Like all human behavior, sexual behavior is socially constructed; even though sex "feels private," sexuality is socially embedded.[16] Moreover, the social construction of sexuality is inevitably linked with cultural concepts of femininity and masculinity. As Dixon-Mueller (1993) clearly synthesized, sexuality and gender are "interlocking domains"; ideas about what constitutes the essence of "maleness" and "femaleness" are expressed in sexual norms and ideologies.

These norms regarding sexuality and gender take different forms. One of them is the "double sexual standard," in which men initiate sexual life earlier than women, are more oriented to enjoyment of the physical aspects of sex, have more sexual partners, and are more likely to have sex outside of marriage. Another is the dual female stereotype (bad girl/whore, good girl/madonna) that depicts "good women" as those ignorant about sex and passive in sexual interactions. Men, in contrast, are expected to be experts on sexuality and have no problem asking for and finding pleasure in sex. Norms that label interpartner communication on sex taboo (especially if initiated by women) or that associate condoms with "illicit sex," are also part of the cultural scenario of almost every society.

In this section we describe how cultural norms of sexuality and gender affect STD prevention and treatment. (Even when, for conciseness, we refer to the "gender barrier," we are referring to the interlocking domains of sexuality and gender.)

Research findings in a wide variety of countries indicate that gender stereotypes and power relations between men and women play a key role in persons' ability to consider themselves at risk for STDs or HIV/AIDS and, therefore, to adopt "safer sex" (see, among others, de Zalduondo and Bernard, 1995; Martin et al., n.d.; Rao Gupta and Weiss, 1993; Caravano, 1995). In other words, there is a broad consensus that gender is a significant barrier to HIV/AIDS prevention and, more generally, to STD prevention, diagnosis, and treatment.

Thus, we intend to "un-pack" and discuss the "gender/sexuality issue," which elsewhere in the literature tends to be treated in an overly schematic way (by assertions like "men always refuse condom use," "women's lack of negotiation skills is the problem," "women do not object to condom use," and so on).

Like other "master statuses" (such as age, race, education), gender organizes a person's understanding of the social world and, particularly, his or her very understanding of sexuality. Gender is also closely associated with the scripts to which people are exposed, the types of choices perceived as viable and legitimate, and the costs and benefits associated with these choices (Laumann et al., 1994). Through these mechanisms, gender norms, power, and stereotypes affect the ability to conceive, propose, and/or adopt effective conduct to prevent and treat STDs.

Paraphrasing Paiva, we could say that "safer sex" confronts the most basic notions of masculinity and femininity: Condom use confronts the most basic notions of male virility—that being a man means 'naturally' having less control over sexual and aggressive impulses, and feeling them more strongly than does a woman. To wear a condom, to be rational, to control sexual drives or take a woman partner's needs into consideration, is to betray maleness. Being a woman is 'naturally' to be more fragile, less aggressive and to be able to control sexual drives. It means being ignorant about sex until marriage, and then to give in to her husband's impulses (Paiva, 1993, 100). As several authors have pointed out, proposing or carrying condoms may imply that a woman is sexually active or looking for sex, connotations that may contradict socially accepted norms by which women must be sexually passive. In addition, economic dependence on men may make it difficult for women to insist on mutual fidelity or condom use (WHO, 1993).

Basically, these arguments hold true for the low-income population in our study. Nevertheless, we intend to show that the process is not straightforward, as our fieldwork made evident a certain pluralism of values and norms regarding gender roles and sexuality. In the context of our study, gender norms and stereotypes, operating in close relation with some popular views about STDs (ideas of contagion, prevention, consequences of STDs, and so on) strongly impinged on risk perception. As discussed previously, the idea that STDs were diseases transmitted by "street women"—or, more vaguely, by "women"—had broad consensus, particularly among male interviewees. Some even considered men's sexuality more vulnerable than women's to STDs. This belief, stemming from the idea that *"la pudrición"* inhibits men from having sex or makes it extremely painful, but does not affect women to the same extent,[17] was quite popular. Such "male weakness" strongly contrasted with women's strong flux, frequently mentioned, along with menstrual blood, as a source of contagion. Female genitals were explicitly referred to as "the hidden," and on several occasions men expressed doubt of women's ability to identify whether they had an STD. Men also showed concern about the possibility of a woman concealing this information from her partner. Phrases like "You can tell when a man has an STD, but not a woman" or "Women may look clean but . . ." were expressed by several interviewees. Male suspiciousness—and female suspiciousness regarding men's fidelity—is part of a sex/gender system characterized by ambivalence and hostility.[18]

The above ideas evoke Petchesky's words (1984), "one senses that where sex is at issue, the male of the species is still regarded by a patriarchal culture and medicine as the delicate and vulnerable one,"[19] and suggest that risk awareness may be high among men. Paradoxically, this is not the case. In the local culture, the dual female image and the stereotypes about masculinity (that men are fearless, horny, and prisoners of a "boy-scout sexuality") counterbalance male perceptions of vulnerability in two ways: first, by inhibiting men's readiness to protect themselves since "A real man takes risks"; second, by preventing them from missing any opportunity for a sexual encounter. The following testimonies illustrate widely-spread notions among men:

You just have to do it [have sex], if the woman is willing. (Male, age 20)

If you are too horny, you may make a mistake. (Male, age 26)

A man goes ahead and does it anyway. "I am a man, and I do it," he says to himself. (Male, age 43)

Hair was meant to be combed [a somewhat vulgar remark to the effect that "wherever there's a woman, you have to do it"]. (Male, age 33)

These beliefs and attitudes coexisted with what some men viewed as ways to protect themselves, such as not having sex or using condoms with certain women ("street women" or those with tattoos).

Women, in turn, felt quite vulnerable. With a few exceptions,[20] the great majority considered men "naturally" unfaithful and women consequently at risk of STDs/HIV. Some even said they worried more about "the plague" than about being deceived. In spite of this awareness, they did not consider the possibility of proposing "safer sex" to their partners.[21] Some did not think it necessary ("[since] you know him") and others declared they did not dare. In the end, fears regarding male reaction (including the chance of a man feeling mistrusted)—and shame—were the main reasons women avoided coping with risk awareness.[22] Married women did, however, conceive of some preventive strategies—expecting husbands to use condoms in secondary relations, or using female condoms themselves. The latter did not seem a very realistic option, however, since female condoms were expensive, men tended not to agree to their use, and the women feared they could not put them in correctly. Nevertheless, the fact that women took these alternatives into consideration may support the argument that they do feel at risk.

To sum up, borrowing Pollak's categories (1992), we could say that the women in our study tended to think in terms of "protection strategies" while the men tended to think in terms of "selection [of partners] strategies."

Turning to a closely related issue, prevention of STDs entails changes in sexual behavior and in eroticism. Given that the only method of reducing the risk of STDs/HIV for sexually active people was, for the study population, the male condom,[23] prevention depended largely on men's acceptance of condom use. The majority of male interviewees were reluctant to use condoms, even though many referred to having used them, or to using them to avoid unwanted pregnancies; men complained about loss of pleasure and interference with the sexual dynamic. Even men who eventually acknowledged never having used condoms repeated the "loss of sensation" argument. Some men also indicated they did not use condoms because for them it was very important to leave their semen inside the vagina.

Many of the women, particularly the older ones, had little or no experience with condoms. Nevertheless, many seemed to place little value on them. Female arguments against condoms took different emphases, in interviews and in focus groups. In face-to-face-interviews, women used arguments similar to those of the men (for example, that condoms interfered with pleasure, prevented feeling the semen inside during intercourse, made them feel "distant"); some women also mentioned that condoms were usually associated with "illicit sex." In the group discussions, however, women most commonly mentioned fear that the condom would break during sexual intercourse or fear that it would cause itching or burning.[24]

In both interviews and group sessions, women indicated that negotiating condom use in stable relationships would be highly problematic. Some also indicated that teenagers of both sexes tended to accept condoms more easily, and that if younger or single, they themselves probably would request eventual partners to use condoms.

Finally, we will briefly discuss the impact of sexuality and gender norms on seeking, and complying with, STDs treatment. Research findings suggest many women did not seek treatment for STDs because they were unaware of the signs and symptoms or because they accepted vaginal discharge and itching as an inevitable part of womanhood or sexual life. The cultural connotations of STDs as diseases of "women of the street" or "dirty women" (as well as fear or shame of being classified "unfaithful" or "deceived") may also have affected the women's ability to recognize symptoms and seek out proper care. The study further revealed that some women had difficulties complying with treatment, particularly when given ovules (considered uncomfortable to insert, not very effective, etc.). Several women indicated their partners would not comply with treatment (usually pills, injections, and sexual abstinence or protected intercourse); only one woman referred to a successful negotiation episode. Men's failure to comply with STD treatment was also referred to by male interviewees; it is worth noting that, although men did consult doctors and follow instructions when they themselves had *"la pudrición,"* they showed little compliance when the STD was diagnosed in their partners.

Final Remarks

We have tried to analyze a complex set of dimensions that must be addressed to understand people's ideas and behavior regarding STDs and to enhance their ability to prevent and treat these diseases. We have talked about knowledge and beliefs, meanings, feelings, social norms, sexuality, and gender stereotypes. Some issues have been covered more deeply than others, and links among domains still need fine-tuning. Nevertheless, we hope to have shown the value of a comprehensive approach, one that takes into consideration lay notions of health and illness, but also cultural scenarios of sexuality, gender, ans interpersonal relations. Our coverage of these cultural domains has varied; stress has been put on lay beliefs regarding STDs.

Exploring what people know and believe about STDs/HIV from an emic perspective was one main concern, since this issue had been only touched on, in this context, before. Our study conclusively indicates that people do have ideas about STDs and that these ideas—which undoubtedly need to be better understood—differ greatly from the biomedical perspective. A great variation in level of knowledge about STDs was observed, with men and the more educated women being better informed. Lay beliefs regarding these illnesses proved strongly tinted by deeply rooted ideas about body fluids—ideas that require better understanding. Although there were variations in the amount and quality of individuals' information on HIV/AIDS, this information seemed more homogeneous than that on STDs.

We also explored how gender relations, and norms of appropriate sexual and nonsexual behavior in relations between men and women, affected individuals' willingness and ability to prevent and treat STDs. Regarding these domains, deeper exploration of gender power relations and of the affective dimension of sexual behavior is necessary.

In addition, the intrapsychic level needs to be addressed in depth. Exploration of what Crawford called "identity work" seems a promising avenue:

Identity work (protecting or reformulating self-boundaries, reinforcing images or reimagining the other) is required of people as they respond to fears of contagion and stigma, as they adopt strategies to protect themselves from *implication*, that is, symbolic connection to "infected" others and the negative characteristics ascribed to them. It is also demanded of people as they make decisions about their own sexuality and sexual behavior and as they respond to the infection of friends and family members. (Crawford, 1994, 1348)

In spite of the limitations of our study, our research findings have provided cues for health promotion and education. First, the data showed how essential it is to take into account ideas from the three cultural domains involved in the STDs field—health and illness, gender, and sexual norms (and the symbolic load of these diseases)—to design comprehensive health promotion and education activities and messages.

In the population studied, young people and adults of both sexes should be provided basic information about their reproductive system and genitals, including characteristics and functions of genital fluids. Regarding STDs, efforts should aim to clarify that most are sexually transmitted while some may be caused by overgrowth of vaginal organisms or be associated with unhygienic personal practices. It should also be emphasized that, whatever the origin, the fact that these diseases are transmitted through sexual intercourse makes protection (in particular, condom use) and prompt and "collaborative" treatment imperative. People must also be informed that women are more susceptible to these infections than men and more likely to suffer from complications of untreated STDs. Both sexes should be made aware that having an STD greatly increases the risk of contracting HIV, and that STDs are frequently asymptomatic, particularly in the case of women, and that even though symptoms may be present in only one partner, treatment should be undergone, in almost all cases, by both.

Regarding HIV/AIDS, the distinction between *being HIV positive* and *having AIDS* is still unclear, and its understanding must be improved. This will contribute to dissipating many misconceptions—

such as the idea that only people with AIDS transmit the disease—
that directly affect willingness and ability to adopt preventive behaviors.

As noted above, transmission of information must go hand in hand
with discussion of sexuality norms and gender stereotypes that allows
the emergence and processing of emotions, prejudices, and doubts.
De-stigmatizing STDs is an essential part of the message. Providing
men and women with opportunities for separate group interactions
seems a necessary first step towards promoting communication of
these matters between partners.

On the basis of this study, we agree with Campbell (1995, 198)
when she states "Men should be targeted directly as a group of male
sex partners, rather than through women." Sensitizing men to the
importance of using condoms in secondary relations may be culturally
appropriate, and seems a better strategy, both practically and strate-
gically, than putting the emphasis on improving women's negotiation
skills, particularly in the case of married women.

Training programs using male peer counselors could be a strategy
to reach men; it has frequently been described in the literature as
successful. Our experience with focus groups suggests this alternative
ought to be evaluated very carefully with key informants. Both young
and adult men in our focus groups underlined that the presence of
an "outsider" as group coordinator enabled them to talk candidly, as
he helped to neutralize the atmosphere of competition and exhibi-
tionism characterizing male interaction when talking about sexual
matters.

Advantage should be taken of the fact that men seek the advice of
doctors and/or pharmacists when they perceive something wrong in
their genitals and presume they have an STD. It would be beneficial
to focus also on physicians and pharmacists, to persuade them of the
importance of transforming the clinical encounter into an opportunity
to discuss with men the importance of reproductive health and their
responsibility in safe sex planning. To develop such a strategy, preliminary work with physicians, aimed at helping them become aware of
lay notions of STDs and of their own gender stereotypes, would be
advisable.[25]

The content of condom promotion messages may have to rely heavily on the condom's benefits as a contraceptive, since men and women
alike expressed negative opinions about the pill and its secondary

effects, and since condom use to avoid unwanted pregnancies is seen as legitimate by men in both stable and casual relationships. As Rao Gupta and Weiss indicate (1995), face-to-face education and mass media campaigns that destigmatize the condom and weaken its association with illicit sex are greatly needed. Also, making the female condom available through health centers deserves further study, given women's positive attitude towards it.

Finally, regular STDs screening procedures during prenatal or family planning visits could help to identify asymptomatic STDs. But, for this to succeed, physicians must also be sensitized to the importance of diagnosing these diseases, a frequently neglected area in their clinical practice. Other problems may arise once this screening procedure has been established; in our study, the local health center and the nearby hospital lacked the required resources to implement appropriate diagnosis and/or to process samples properly and in time. This last point calls attention to service supply and accessibility, key factors in STDs prevention and treatment that also must be addressed with specific interventions to effectively enhance reproductive health.

Helping people to become more conscious of health problems, and consequently to have better chances of taking care of themselves and their partners, has been our focus. To achieve such goals, both the population and the health care system need targeting. We hope to have contributed to the design of culturally appropriate responses to the "silent epidemic."

Acknowledgements

This chapter is based on the results of the project "Psychosocial and Cultural Factors in the Prevention and Treatment of STDs: Power, Love, and Pleasure in the Negotiations between Genders," conducted by the authors and Edith A. Pantelides (CENEP-Argentina), and supported by the World Health Organization's Task Force for Social Science Research on Reproductive Health.

Notes

1. We conducted ten focus groups: three with young men age eighteen to twenty-five, three with young women, two with adult men age twenty-five to fifty, and two with adult women, as well as twenty in-depth interviews with the same target population.

2. Fitzpatrick et al. (1984) emphasize "people may be quite uncomfortable about expressing and organizing ideas which normally remain tacit
background resources to be drawn upon when coping with their own or
other people's illnesses" (1984, 18). Pill and Scott (1982) describe their respondents as unsure of themselves and less articulate when discussing eti-
ological topics, with the tone of the interviews becoming more hesitant and
statements more often qualified by such phrases as "I suppose."

3. The "emic" perspective is appropriate to capturing the problem from
the subjects' point of view—in the terms of their perceptions and categories
(Pelto and Pelto, 1978).

4. Defining the starting question was a demanding task. We decided to
probe one of the possibilities suggested in the Helitzer-Allen and Allen ethnographic protocol for the study of STDs (1994).

5. Other studies have also confirmed that the popular notion of STDs
differs greatly from the biomedical perspective. In relation to a similar starting question, a study in Haiti revealed that the interviewees included as
STDs some diseases (from the list) that could be transmitted between couples by other means than sexual relations. Some of the mentioned diseases—
like tuberculosis—were conceived as STDs because the close proximity of
the partners during the sexual act could facilitate contagion through cough-
ing (Désormeaux et al., 1992).

6. There is much contradictory evidence as to which STD the popular
expression "rotting" refers. On the one hand, some key informants contend
the term alludes to syphilis; "rotting" or "to be rotted" are the words most
often used to describe syphilis, the most well-known in popular experience
(Dominguez Mon, 1991). On the other hand, the symptoms attributed to
"rotting" and the short time taken, it was said, for the symptoms to appear,
suggest that the subjects might have been referring to gonorrhea or chla-
mydia infection (Helitzer-Allen and Allen, 1994).

7. These differences were conspicuously evident in the focus groups.

8. It is worth noting that seven of the ten women individually interviewed wanted to make clear that they had never had an STD. Expressions
like "It didn't happen to me," "I never had it," were repeatedly mentioned.
The women also stated, more often than the men, that they had no friends,
acquaintances, or relatives who had any of these diseases. The same reactions
held for women in the focus groups. In contrast, only two of the ten men
participating in the in-depth interviews stated that they had never had diseases of this kind; the majority of participants in the focus groups admitted
to having experienced, and to knowing of friends or acquaintances with, the
problem.

9. The cultural significance of menstruation as a polluted, or a purifying,
agent has been explored in different cultures (Skultans, 1970; Ngubane,
1977; Snow and Johnson, 1977; Martin, 1992; and Fachel, 1995, and others).
We did not systematically explore the cultural meanings of menstruation in

this study. However, in other research developed with the same target population, there was seen a widespread belief among women that menstruation is a purification and cleansing process through which the organism rids itself of impurities (Balán and Ramos, 1989).

10. In some languages these diseases are even labeled as "women's diseases," or characterized as infections that "good" men catch from "bad" women (McCormack, 1982).

11. Speaking about the "environmental route" of STD transmission, analogies with cholera were repeatedly reported, emphasizing the "unclean-related view" of the STD threat.

12. We carried out a very small number of interviews with doctors, whom we addressed as key informants. Their testimonies indicate that doctors may be reinforcing many lay notions. As we were told, to "protect the family," vague answers to questions about STD transmission are frequently given—referring, for instance, only to the importance of hygiene.

13. This difficulty has also been confirmed in studies in other countries, such as Brazil (Vasconcelos et al., 1993) and Uganda (Obbo, 1991).

14. The profound emotional load of STDs calls for an empathetic response by medical counselors, but they have not been trained to deal with such complex issues.

15. Women were also very enthusiastic about the female condom, but it did not seem a practical strategy for them.

16. Kinship and family systems, sexual regulations and definitions of communities, national and world systems—each and all simultaneously set the external limits on sexual experience and shape individual and group behavior (Ross and Rapp, 1983).

17. In one male focus group, however, some participants expressed the idea that women with "rotting" may suffer more than men during sexual intercourse.

18. Generally speaking, men tended to blame women, describing them as dirty, over-demanding, and too smart/"*vivas.*" Women, in turn, considered men irresponsible, cold, naturally unfaithful. Women regretted their share in the sexual division of labor and complained of not having the same freedom as men.

19. The statement stemmed from the fact that researchers and male subjects were extremely concerned about the possibilities of the "undesirable side effects" that chemical contraceptives could cause in men.

20. Some women explicitly defined themselves as "nice women" or "women of the home" (*señora de su casa*), and believed that their status protected them from the risk of STDs.

21. Only three young women of the sixty interviewed declared that they would not have sex without a condom.

22. A small number of assertive women challenged the others to protect themselves, arguing that a loving husband would care for their health.

23. The female condom was just beginning to be known among our population.

24. The more intimate climate of the interview may have encouraged women to refer more openly to eroticism, thus explaining the difference from testimonies collected in group sessions.

25. Even though we carried out very few interviews with doctors, our evidence suggests that gender stereotypes also affect physicians' ability to diagnose STDs and to give clear and effective instructions for prevention and treatment.

References

Balán, J., and Ramos, S. (1989). "La Medicalización del Comportamiento Reproductivo: Un Estudio de los Sectores Populares Urbanos." *Documentos CEDES* 29. Buenos Aires.

Becker, M., and Maiman, L. (1983). "Models of Health-Related Behavior." In Mechanic, D. (ed.), *Handbook of Health, Health Care, and the Health Professions*. New York: Free Press.

Benería, L., and Roldán, M. (1992). *Las Encrucijadas de Clase y Género: Trabajo a Domicilio, Subcontratación y Dinámica de la Unidad Doméstica en la Ciudad De México*. Mexico City: El Colegio de México-FCE.

Campbell, C. (1995). "Male Gender Roles and Sexuality: Implications for Women's AIDS Risk and Prevention." *Social Science and Medicine*, 41, no. 2.

Caravano, K. (1995). "VIH/SIDA y los Desafios que Enfrentan los Hombres: Implicaciones para un Cambio de Conducta." DESIDAMOS, Año 3. No. 1.

Cleary, P. (1988). "Education and the Prevention of AIDS." *Law, Medicine, and Health Care*, 16(3/4):267–73.

Crawford, R. (1994). "The Boundaries of Self and the Unhealthy Other: Reflections on Health, Culture, and AIDS." *Social Science and Medicine*, 38(10):1347–65.

Désormeaux, J. et al. (1992). "The Importance of Local Concepts of Contagion and Sexual Conduct for AIDS Education: A Case from Urban Haiti. (Mimeographed).

de Zalduondo, B. O., and Bernard, J. M. (1995) "Meanings and Consequences of Sexual-Economic Exchange: Gender, Poverty, and Sexual Risk Behavior in Urban Haiti." In Parker, R. G., and Gagnon, J. (eds.), *Conceiving Sexuality: Approaches to Sex Research in a Postmodern World*, 157–80. New York and London: Routledge.

Dixon-Mueller, R. (1993). "The Sexuality Connection in Reproductive Health." *Studies in Family Planning*, 24, no. 5.

Dixon-Mueller, R., and Wasserheit, J. (1991). *The Culture of Silence. Reproductive Tract Infection among Women in the Third World*. New York: IWHC.

Dominguez Mon, A. (1991). "La Construcción Social de Estigmas: El Caso de las ETS in la Atención Hospitalaria." Mimeographed.

Fachel, O. (1995). "Sangue, Fertilidade, e Práticas Contraceptivas." In Fachel, O. (ed.), *Corpo e Significado: Ensaios de Antropologia Social*. Porto Alegre: Editora da Universidade.

Fitzpatrick, R., et al. (eds.) (1984). *The Experience of Illness*. London: Tavistock.

Freidson, E. (1978). *La Profesión Médica: Un Estudio de Sociología del Conocimiento Aplicado*. Barcelona: Península.

Gagnon, J. (1988). "Sex Research and Sexual Conduct in the Era of AIDS." *Journal of Acquired Immune Deficiency Syndromes*, 1: 593–601.

———. (1990). "The Explicit and Implicit Use of the Scripting Perspective in Sex Research." *Annual Review of Sex Research*, 1: 1–43.

Giddens, A. (1992). *The Transformation of Intimacy: Sexuality, Love, and Eroticism in Modern Societies*. Stanford: Stanford University Press.

Giele, J. (1988). *Gender and Sex Roles*. London: Sage.

Helitzer-Allen, D., and Allen, H. (1994). *The Manual for Targeted Intervention Research on Sexually Transmitted Illnesses with Community Members*. Baltimore: AIDSCAP.

Hochbaum, G. M. (1981). "Behavior Change as the Goal of Health Education." *Eta Sigma Gamman*, 3–6.

Laumann, E., et al. (1994). *The Social Organization of Sexuality: Sexual Practices in the United States*. Chicago: University of Chicago Press.

Loyola, A. (1994). "AIDS e Prevençao da AIDS no Rio de Janeiro." In Loyola, A. (ed.), *AIDS e Sexualidade: O Ponto de Vista das Ciencias Humanas*. Rio de Janeiro: Relume-Dumará.

Martin, D., Barbosa, R. M., and Villela, W. [n.d.]. "Mulher, Sexualidade, e Prevençao da AIDS." Mimeographed.

Martin, E. (1992). *The Women in the Body: A Cultural Analysis of Reproduction*. Boston: Beacon Press.

McCormack, W. (1982). "Sexually Transmitted Diseases: Women as Victims." *The Journal of the American Medical Association*, 248(2).

Mechanic, D. (1978). *Medical Sociology: A Comprehensive Text*. New York: Free Press.

Ngubane, H. (1977). *Body and Mind in Zulu Medicine*. London: Academic Press.

Obbo, C. (1991). "HIV Transmission: Men are the Solution. A Ugandan Perspective." Paper presented at the conference Consequences of HIV/AIDS in Eastern Africa, Washington, DC, 14–19 February.

Paiva, V. (1993). "Sexuality, Condom Use, and Gender Norms among Brazilian Teenagers." *Reproductive Health Matters*, no. 2.

Parker, R. G. (1992). "Sexual Diversity, Cultural Analysis and AIDS Education in Brazil." In Herdt, G., and Lindenbaum, S., (eds.), *The Time of*

AIDS: Social Analysis, Theory, and Method, 225–42. Newbury Park, CA.: Sage Publications.

Pelto, P., and Pelto, G. (1978). "Units of Observation: Emic and Etic Approaches." In *Anthropological Research: The Structure of Inquiry*. Cambridge: Cambridge University Press.

Petchesky, R. (1984). *Abortion and Woman's Choice: The State, Sexuality, and Reproductive Freedom*. Boston: Northeastern University Press.

Pill, R., and Scott, N. C. H. (1982). "Concepts of Illness Causation and Responsibility: Some Preliminary Data from a Sample of Working-Class Mothers." *Social Science and Medicine*, 16(1):43–52.

Pollak, M. (1992). "Understanding Sexual Behaviour and Its Change." In Pollak, M., Paicheler, G., and Pierret, J. (eds.), *AIDS: A Problem for Sociological Research*, 40(3):85–102.

Rao Gupta, G., and Weiss, E. (1993). *Women and AIDS: Developing a New Health Strategy*. ICRW Policy Series.

———. (1995). "Women's Lives and Sex: Implications for AIDS Prevention." In Parker, R. G., and Gagnon, J. (eds), *Conceiving Sexuality: Approaches to Sex Research in a Postmodern World*, 259–70. New York and London: Routledge.

Rosenstock, I. M. (1960). "What Research in Motivation Suggests for Public Health." *American Journal of Public Health*, 50:295–301.

———. (1966). "Why People Use Health Services." *Milbank Memorial Fund Quarterly*, 44:94–124.

Rosenstock, I. M., and Becker, M. (1974). "Social Learning Theory and the Health Belief Model." *Health Education Quarterly*, 15:175–83.

Rosenstock, I. M., and Kirscht, J. P. (1974). "The Health Belief Model and Personal Health Behavior." *Health Education Monographs*, 2:470–73

Ross, E., and Rapp, R. (1983). "Sex and Society: A Research Note from Social History and Anthropology." Snitow, A., Stansell, C., and Thompson, S., (eds.), *Powers of Desire*. New York: Monthly Review Press.

Rubin, G. (1992). "El Placer y el Peligro: Hacia una Política de la Sexualidad." In Vance, C. S. (ed.), *Placer y Peligro: Explorando la Sexualidad Femenina*, 113–90, Madrid: Editora Revolución.

Skultans, V. (1970). "The Symbolic Significance of Menstruation and Menopause." *Man*, 5:639–51.

Snow, L. F., and Johnson, S. M. (1977). "Modern Day Menstrual Folklore." *Journal of the American Medical Association*, 237:2736–2739.

Suchman, E. A. (1965). "Stages of Illness and Medical Care." *Journal of Health and Social Behavior*, 6:114–28.

Vasconcelos, A. et al. (1993). *AIDS and Sexuality among Low-Income Adolescent Women in Recife, Brazil*. Washington, DC: ICRW.

World Health Organization, Global Programme on AIDS. (1993). "Sexual Negotiation, the Empowerment of Women, and the Female Condom: General Protocol." Mimeographed.

Part Three

Hegemony, Oppression, and Empowerment

Chapter Seven

AIDS, Medicine, and Moral
Panic in the Philippines

Michael L. Tan

Little has been written about how the AIDS epidemic in developing
countries has affected discourse on sex and sexuality, and, more important, how such discourse reflects persistence as well as change in
sexual ideologies. In this paper, I will describe popular representations
of sex and sexuality in relation to the emerging AIDS epidemic in the
Philippines. I will draw mainly from reports in the broadsheets—large
circulation daily newspapers that cater mainly to the middle- and
high-income groups (as opposed to tabloids, which also have large
circulations but have fewer pages and are cheaper, catering to low-
income groups). Since the broadsheets are aimed toward elite or
dominant social groups, they are important in reflecting, as well as
shaping, public policy. In addition, using the broadsheets—which are
in English—allows me to move into public policy documents, which
are also in English. This class bias in the selection of broadsheets is
intentional, because I wish to focus my analysis on the ideological
messages in these representations, and to show the many instances of
interface between sexual and class ideologies in what can be characterized as moral panic.

Let me begin by quoting at length from Cohen's pioneering work:

Societies appear to be subject, every now and then, to periods of moral panic.
A condition, episode, person or group of persons emerges to become defined
as a threat to societal values and interests; its nature is presented in a stylized
and stereotypical fashion by the mass media; the moral barricades are
manned by editors, bishops, politicians and other right-thinking people; socially accredited experts pronounce their diagnoses and solutions; ways of
coping are evolved or (more often) resorted to; the condition then disappears, submerges or deteriorates and becomes more visible. Sometimes the
object of the panic is quite novel and at other times . . . suddenly appears in

the limelight. Sometimes the panic passes over and is forgotten, except in folklore and collective memory; at other times it has more serious and long-lasting repercussions and might produce such changes as those in legal and social policy or even in the way the society conceives itself. (Cohen, 1972:9)

Cohen's description is particularly useful for examining the social framework of what have often become clichés in the literature on HIV/AIDS, gender, and sexuality: misogyny, homophobia, and xenophobia. I shall look at how HIV/AIDS is itself socially constructed (and reconstructed) in the exchange between "medical" and "lay" sectors, and how the moral barricades created in AIDS discourses draw power and legitimacy from medicine.

As Parker points out, part of the modernization of sexual life generally seems to involve processes in which "the moral discourses of social hygiene and modern medicine have themselves been extended and transformed" (Parker, 1991:85–87). Understanding the social and historical context of this transformation is important, especially in this age of HIV and AIDS.

Urban Myths and HIV Fugitives

I would like to start by presenting a sampling of stories that have appeared in the media. These stories are selected because they were not one-time features; they have taken on a life of their own, and gained prominence before fading from fickle public memory. Even afterwards, we find lingering traces that at times reappear, much like moral panic. The earliest of these urban myths first appeared in 1988 and is recounted, a year later, by Antonio Abaya, a Filipino journalist: "The most celebrated AIDS carrier in Philippine medical history so far was the pretty Brazilian heterosexual houri who romped with more than one hundred macho Filipinos before she was arrested and deported. She has probably infected more Filipinos than the entire U.S. Seventh Fleet and Thirteenth Air Force combined" (*Business World*, August 15, 1989).

It does not matter that no one has ever proven a single case of infection from this Brazilian woman; in fact, there are no records or photographs of her. Beginning in 1994, we find a proliferation of such stories in the newspapers, in spite (or perhaps, I suspect, because) of the intensification of AIDS awareness campaigns. The stories began with that of Sarah Jane Salazar, first of what I shall call "HIV/AIDS fugitives," targets of often vicious media reports and, at times, even of police hunts. But I shall return later to Sarah Jane, since her story has become a saga.

For now I shall make a quick leap to September 1994, when articles began to appear claiming that popular actor Richard Gomez had left the country to be treated for AIDS. The articles claimed that Gomez, a macho heartthrob, had acquired HIV from a gay relationship. A furious Gomez, who had in fact gone abroad to attend a film course, flew home and had a highly publicized "AIDS test," with the result issued on the spot, with no less than the Health Secretary proclaiming the actor HIV-negative.

Gomez's case stands in stark contrast to an incident that erupted only a month later. In October 1994, Paterno Menzon, a congressman from Northern Samar, fed reports to the press about two female prostitutes who had infected "at least forty-seven prominent individuals in Northern Samar." One newspaper report gave this detailed account: "Two 'very sexy and beautiful' prostitutes who were driven out of Olongapo City when the U.S. naval base in that place was closed down went to Northern Samar and allegedly infected with AIDS at least forty-seven prominent businessmen and politicians in the province" (*Today*, October 6, 1994).

The congressman called on the two women to come forward and be tested, "Prudence indicates that they should submit themselves to HIV tests for their own good." Menzon claimed: "One of the two HIV-infected female commercial sex workers was said to have enrolled as a nursing student in a university in the province. She also worked as a singer in a nightclub in Catarman . . . The woman is suspected of having infected influential men in Northern Samar, and of keeping a diary that lists the names of her clients."

One of the women later surfaced to deny the allegations. Her impoverished family had to find ways to get her to Manila to be tested, and a small news item ultimately "cleared" her. The congressman became the target of criticism in the press for a brief period before the issue faded. No one ever pursued the case of the other woman.

I move now to another story. In November 1994, Dr. Rene Bullecer of AIDS-Free Philippines was featured in the newspapers claiming that seventeen Filipinos on a Panamanian ship had been found to have AIDS. Bullecer said the seventeen Filipinos were part of "a crew of thirty-nine who all tested positive for HIV." He said this was the third time Filipino seamen had been found to "have AIDS," the first being in 1991 when twenty-five seamen were found positive, the second in 1992 when three tested positive. "Although their identities could not be immediately known," he said, "the seventeen Filipinos are all in their early twenties, single, and were connected with the Panamanian-registered cargo vessel for at least a year." Bullecer would not give a ship name, simply stating, "It was a cargo ship cruising around the world." He said he was certain the seamen had been infected with the virus during a stopover in either Africa or Brazil, "where AIDS cases are high." It could not be possible, he added, that they got the disease in the Philippines since all overseas contract workers undergo HIV testing before being permitted to leave the country (*Inquirer*, November 17, 1994). Bullecer's seamen stories continue to circulate among Filipinos, and in December 1995, while in Rotterdam, I even heard the story—with different figures—from a group helping Filipino seamen.

Bullecer's group (AIDS-Free Philippines), supported by the Roman Catholic church, goes around claiming that condoms do not work against HIV. This particular story was actually atypical for Bullecer, in that most of his stories focus on "hospitality girls," a euphemism for female sex workers; an early example of this genre was a November 13, 1989, *Newsday* article, "10 AIDS Carriers Reported Missing," which claimed that health authorities "have intensified the hunt for ten hospitality girls who have disappeared after testing positive for AIDS antibodies," and further asserted, "two of these girls went abroad. Their destination, however, is unknown." This article was about Angeles City, where in 1995, amid reports of a resurgence of prostitution in the area, newspapers reported on "thirty-three missing HIV-positive prostitutes, including two of whom have developed AIDS" (*Philippine Daily Inquirer*, July 6, 1995). The most recent example is a tabloid article entitled "13 Cavite Bar Girls HIV Carriers" (*People's Journal Tonight*, March 27, 1996), which states that thirteen women were isolated after having been found HIV-positive. The "source" of the infection was said to be a Filipino who had been in the U.S. Navy.

Typically, then, urban myths have been built in which women (usually sex workers) or men (usually with hints of their being homosexual) test positive for HIV infection. The women or men then disappear.

Fears are expressed that they may be spreading the virus. Appeals are made for such fugitives to turn themselves in and even to take another test "for their own good."

The case of Sarah Jane Salazar is perhaps the longest-running of this genre. In 1994, a former movie gossip columnist turned politician informed the press that there was a "bar girl" who was HIV positive and was now roaming the country. Newspapers reported periodic Sarah Jane sightings. In March, for example, she was reported in Cotobato City, in the southern Philippines, where she was said to be "running away from armed men who wanted to kill her to prevent the spread of the killer disease" (*Manila Chronicle*, March 17, 1994). Reporters also tried to reconstruct Sarah Jane's past. In March, the health department ordered the testing of 1,050 prisoners in Muntin-lupa, the national penitentiary, because of rumors that "seventy-eight prisoners had been possible former clients of an AIDS-afflicted prostitute," referring to Sarah Jane (*Star*, March 19, 1994).

Sarah Jane eventually surfaced, ironically under the "protection" of the movie-columnist politician who had first "outed" her. Together with her patron, she appeared at a press conference with the health secretary, who said she was going to be part of the health department's team of AIDS educators. A movie has since been made about Sarah, and through the years, she has continued to provide material for newspapers. In 1995, one tabloid ran the headline "I Don't Bite," following reports that Sarah Jane had bitten a neighbor in a fight; reporters speculated whether she could infect people with HIV. More recently, a newspaper article headlined "Sarah Jane Feared Infecting Youths" stated: "The guardian of self-confessed AIDS victim Sarah Jane Salazar yesterday asked the Department of Health to confine the girl in one of the department's AIDS centers to stop her from continuing sexual activities" (*Manila Chronicle*, February 7, 1995). And the basis for this guardian's fears? Sarah Jane was reported to stay out until "around one to four A.M."

Historical Retrospectives: from U.S. Bases
to *Balikbayans*

There is much to analyze in the content of the urban myths, but we should first reflect briefly on the origins of some of these representations.

The first media-reported cases of HIV in the Philippines date to about 1985. Most involved female sex workers from bars in Angeles and Subic, rest and recreation areas for U.S. military bases. For some time, the *Kano* (short for Americano) were blamed for AIDS, fanning the strong anti-U.S.-bases sentiment that meshed with the anti-Marcos movement. GABRIELA, a militant women's organization, produced posters reading "No Bases, No Nukes, No AIDS." Marcos fell in 1986, and the bases were eventually removed in 1992, but perceptions of a foreign "carrier" remain strong; in my research with both female and male sex workers, the "safer sex" options are often dropped when the customer is Filipino. There are also varying perceptions about risk; other Asians are generally seen as "clean," while Europeans and Americans are perceived as riskier.

While few Africans ever visit the Philippines, it is interesting to see how the West's media coverage has shaped Filipino perceptions, drawing on the anti-black racism in the country. For example, Antonio Abaya, a respected journalist, had two long articles on AIDS in his column in a business newspaper. Abaya said his information was based on a visiting American medical researcher. Note the use of medical statistics mixed with racist lore, drawn both from local and international sources:

Because of non-reporting and inefficiency in many African countries, the figures for the Dark Continent are only estimates.

He [the medical researcher] calculates that by mid-2000, if no cure is found, Congo's present two million inhabitants will have been totally infected or dead.

Both the U.S. and Switzerland are "up there" (in AIDS figures) probably because of the efficiency of their data gathering. Or because of exceptionally large homosexual and/or drug addict populations. Additionally, the US is about 18 percent Black.

The apparent predisposition or weak resistance of the Black race to the HIVirus [sic] is evident, for example, in heavily Black Brazil, which in 1989 had an AIDS case rate of 44.5 per one million, while predominantly white neighbors Argentina and Uruguay had 9.8 and 15.1 respectively.

It is interesting to note that the association between HIV and homosexuals, although present, does not dominate media representations. Conservative religious groups occasionally point out that HIV "mainly" affects homosexuals, but cite figures from the West. And when health officials ordered testing of inmates in Muntinlupa prison, several newspapers also referred to "gay" inmates: "Hundreds of convicts here serving lifetime jail terms, including eighteen confirmed homosexuals, have voluntarily submitted themselves to a Department of Health (DOH) team extracting blood specimens to check if any of them are afflicted with HIV or suffering from AIDS."

Yet in contrast to the relative lack of press coverage of HIV and homosexuality, homosexual and bisexual men compromise about 20 percent of all reported HIV cases in the Philippines, and about 40 percent of all AIDS cases. This shows that attempts by government and NGOs to de-gay the epidemic have actually been quite successful—which presents both advantages and disadvantages for gay community groups, spared to some extent of public attacks, but also receiving low priority for funding.

This is not to say that homosexuals are not targeted in the moral panic associated with AIDS. As in many countries in the region, the homosexual is, in the public mind, the effeminate cross-dresser, tolerated as a source of entertainment but discriminated against as social deviant. Such perceptions predate AIDS but may have become more powerful in the AIDS era. I will consider such AIDS-related discrimination later in this paper.

Another group occasionally singled out in the media for association with HIV/AIDS are Filipinos who have lived or worked overseas. About twenty percent of reported HIV cases involve *balikbayan* Filipinos, *balikbayan* meaning returnees. An estimated 1.5 million Filipinos are now permanent residents in the United States, and another 4.5 million are classified as overseas contract workers (i.e., people with one- to three-year contracts) in various countries. This includes about 250,000 seafarers and many women working as domestics or in the entertainment industry. This tremendous international movement inevitably impacts both the way HIV spreads in the Philippines and public discourse on HIV. For example, in a recent article about a Filipino with HIV, the reporter notes, "Nick says with a distinctive California twang——" (*Philippine Daily Inquirer*, November 28, 1994). In a sense, this comes full circle, from the early perception of foreigners bringing in HIV to that of Filipinos working overseas and bringing back HIV.

Female sex workers have carried the heaviest burden of being identified with HIV/AIDS. Such perceptions draw on older concepts of

STDs as *sakit ng babae* or women's diseases. We continue to find, even among health professionals, people who believe that these diseases, including HIV, are transmitted more frequently from women to men. Figures from the government's testing program undoubtedly reinforce such perceptions, a point to which I shall return.

To recapitulate, the 1980s concentrated on foreign origins of HIV, while in the 1990s attention has shifted to how HIV is spreading locally. An international context remains, in the representations of seamen and overseas contract workers. What is striking is that all these representations carry a strong "medical" element of subterfuge and massive infection, followed by arrests and/or testing, and sometimes another episode of mysterious disappearances.

Controlling Sexuality

In October 1995, newspapers reported proposals to distribute condoms to Filipino athletes participating in the eighteenth Southeast Asian Games taking place in Thailand. Philippine Sports Commissioner Celso Dayrit is quoted with the following reaction:

Our athletes will go to the SEA Games to compete in their respective sports with their full potential to excel and bring back honors for the country . . . They will do this to the best of their physical and mental abilities for the greater glory of God . . . We should never suggest, allow or condone any other activities that would only disrupt their concentration to excel, much less be an instrument to any illicit or immoral activity. (*Evening Paper*, October 19, 1995)

The images of AIDS are inextricably intertwined with those of sex. As a result, it is not surprising to find AIDS discourse shuttling between sex-related themes—pleasure and danger, discipline and death. Anything "sexual" has to be disruptive, if not dangerous, as exemplified by an early Philippine National Red Cross poster advising the following (because they might have HIV) not to donate blood: homosexuals, bisexuals . . . and heterosexuals. Although the poster is no longer used, some Red Cross chapters have evolved a new way of "assuring" safe blood; men with tattoos and earrings are banned from blood donation.

The fear of sex and sexuality is evident in many public documents.

The following are excerpts from a position paper presented by the Department of Labor during a workshop on AIDS in December 1992:

AIDS is a serious malady. It is associated with irregular or promiscuous sex activities. It is sometimes referred to as a disease of the homosexuals, bisexuals and heterosexuals. Never mind if it can be caused or transmitted by transfusion of infected blood to the sick or the victims of accidents, for example. Or by breastfeeding by HIV infected mother to the child. It is a debilitating and disgraceful disease.

Let us look at another government position paper, this one from the National Bureau of Investigation (NBI). Putting Freud on his head, the paper carries the title "Acquired Immune Deficiency Syndrome: A Disease of the Civilization." The first paragraph describes AIDS as a highly transmissible disease with "symptoms such as intensive susceptibility to pulmonary diseases, dermatological eruptions and deficiencies, and other rapidly debilitating physical and functional conditions of the human body."

The second paragraph elaborates on AIDS as "a disease of the civilization": "AIDS is transmitted as a consequence of sexual and piercing contact with an open membrane of the body by a carrier of the virus. It is a socially-transmitted disease of the civilization which requires prevention rather than treatment."

If indeed the writer was developing his or her thoughts more or less lucidly (though not necessarily logically), we find the following themes: sex, piercing, carrier, virus, disease, civilization, prostitution, pervert (sic) sexual behavior, injection-drug dependence. The consequences of these themes are overwhelming, "dermatological eruptions and deficiencies, and other rapidly debilitating physical and functional conditions of the human body."

It is quite clear how the "medical consequences" are meant to epitomize social disruption: AIDS is an affliction and an eruption. The Department of Labor paper continues with this interesting passage on ignorance and knowledge: "The main reason for the incidence of AIDS is commonly attributed to carelessness about sexual practices and ignorance of the disease. The latter presupposes some knowledge of the disease and use of free will. However, such knowledge can mean ignorance of the terrible consequences of such carelessness."

Knowledge is ignorance. Reading this position paper (admittedly, several times), I think I finally understand the writer(s)'s line of argument (knowledge, ignorance, or free will are irrelevant): Knowledge of sex is always dangerous because it is tantamount to denial of HIV's "terrible consequences." Arguments like this resonate in statements such as those of Max Ricketts, of Pro-Life Philippines, who describes HIV programs of "sex indoctrination, abortifacient drugs, and condom-mania" as developed by "militant homosexuals and brave-new-world secular humanists" (*Manila Bulletin*, February 11, 1994). It is important to pick up on this theme of "secular humanism," a catchword used by conservatives in attacking HIV programs. The theme is not just dangerous sexuality but dangerous sexual knowledge.

It is not surprising that the campaign against HIV education programs is spearheaded by the same groups opposing sex education; this has affected even research. The Health Action Information Network, for example, has been asked twice—appropriately, by a bishop and by a doctor—why we were doing sex research and whether such research wouldn't give young people ideas. Both venerable figures were upset by our questions about with whom people had sex; the doctor said that by asking if people had sex with sex workers, we were suggesting they go have such sex.

These linkages between knowledge and danger are pervasive. For example, one editorial on the problem of STDs was entitled "Reckless Concupiscence" (*Manila Times*, May 26, 1993). The editorial was actually quite supportive of HIV prevention campaigns, including condom use, but the choice of words offered insights into how Catholic catechism classes introduce terms and concepts that have become very much a part of the middle-class Filipino world view.

Policing the Citizenry

What we see now is a montage of images—of a virus and of individuals, of knowledge and of ignorance, and of a reckless concupiscence that needs to be controlled.

I shall return to these calls for individuals to control their sexuality. What I shall discuss now are the themes of control. In the NBI position paper, we find the suggestion to launch "educational," "psychological," and "social" measures against HIV/AIDS. In elaborating on the "social," the paper calls for "thorough cleansing and reinforcement" of "the moral fiber of the people." The paper moves into a litany of social ills, such as "failure of family relations, academic negligence, the degenerating socioeconomic and political conditions prevailing, and the corrupt and graft-laden government systems," which are linked to "the resultant ruin of the moral values of our people, the desperate attitudes and character, and ultimately, the high rise in the incidence of criminality," followed by crimes, such as drug addiction and prostitution, that provide the "major catalysts to the transmission of the AIDS virus." The second part of the NBI paper completes the construction of HIV by linking it to "morality" and "criminality."

"Utak pulis" (literally, police brains), a friend exclaimed upon reading the position paper. *Utak pulis*, in a broader context, is a mind-set, a dominant and dominating ideology in our social and political structures. *Utak pulis* manifests itself in calls for mandatory testing and for quarantine of persons with HIV/AIDS. But it is not enough to attribute these calls to lack of understanding of the medical facts, such as the window period in HIV-antibody testing. We have to recognize that support for mandatory testing and quarantine relate to how HIV/AIDS is equated to immorality and criminality; testing becomes, in fact, surveillance and punishment.

There is a strong religious undercurrent to much of this discourse. In several Health Action Information Network surveys with young adults, including medical and nursing students, many agree with the statement "AIDS is a punishment from God." And in his pastoral letter "Our Christian Approach to AIDS," Cardinal Jaime Sin warned that "Morality does not compel obedience. Morality does not, of its nature, carry external sanctions. But we close our ears to the voice of morality only at our peril."

This religious discourse often contains an image of ruthless divine retribution. If Eve's reckless concupiscence is at the root of our problems, then we must heed the warnings of another woman, the Virgin Mary, much loved in the Philippines. An article appearing in *Business World* (August 15, 1989) features messages from "Our Lady and Our Lord to Veronica Luekens, a seer living in Bayside, Long Island, New York." The message says there have been three plagues from God—Legionnaire's Disease, herpes, and AIDS, and cites Jesus as saying:

My children, I shall not allow the scientific world to find a cure for AIDS because of the horrible nature of what brings in this disease called AIDS. It is being flaunted now as though the good were to be stomped upon and the bad shall receive the glory. Homosexuality shall never be accepted . . . This shall not be accepted nor condoned by the eternal Father even if he has to send another plague upon you. No, my children, they shall not, NOT be given the cure.

Religious groups have pushed for legislation on sex and sexuality, despite Cardinal Sin's assertion that morality carries no external sanctions. Central to this process of social control is the process of segregation, of creating "the other," of constructing "high-risk groups." For example, in "Our Christian Approach to AIDS," the Cardinal starts out by asserting "It is wrong to see AIDS as a scourge willed by God to punish a sinful world," but goes on to propose "When we do not conform to authentic human sexual expression, AIDS becomes a glaring threat. Homosexual activity is immoral due to the inherent impossibility of procreation and the lack of any true physical union." The "deficiency" here comes from lack of "authenticity" and of "true physical union." This immorality justifies sanctions for members of this group and for those pursuing other "deviant practices." It should not be surprising that these conservative groups push hardest to legislate those forms of sex and sexuality lacking such "authenticity," including contraception, abortion, and homosexuality.

We find, then, the construction of the deviant, with AIDS as retribution; in contrast stand that vague mass of people, the "general population." An article appearing on December 3, 1991, is headlined "General Population Now Becoming More Vulnerable to AIDS." The article reports that "eleven potential blood donors" were identified as HIV-positive, but that the health department qualified such blood donors as "low-risk" because they "come from the general population (and) do not usually engage in such risky behavior as prostitution, sex with multiple partners, and use of intravenous drugs." In effect, to describe "high-risk" groups is to construct a "low-risk" general population as well. Many problems arise from this dichotomy, especially in relation to a "low-risk" but "vulnerable" general population. In 1995, health secretary Jaime Galvez Tan announced that some 62,000 Filipinos had HIV, but that there was no cause for panic. The newspapers reported, "He said that most of these anonymous victims be-

long to the high-risk groups such as homosexuals, polygamous heterosexuals, and intravenous drug users" (*Manila Chronicle*, June 16,
1995). Boundaries blurred and fears heightened over these "victims,"
anonymous yet identifiable—for after all, the homosexual and the
polygamous heterosexual were to be found within families, within
neighborhoods. Even the intravenous drug user was close at hand,
for although injecting drug users are a very small population, the idea
of "drug user" evoked young men congregating in neighborhood cor-
ner stores.

As the ominous shadows lengthened, new barricades were needed.
More laws were proposed. In 1992, one member of congress introduced a bill that would create red-light districts throughout the country, to be supervised by the health department, mainly through periodic medical testing of sex workers. The congressman who filed the
bill said he had the support of his bishop. The merging of the roles
of medical guardian and moral guardian could not have been more
graphically constructed.

Medicalizing the Policing

We see that much discourse around HIV/AIDS is a blend of the
medical and the religious. It is clear, however, that with AIDS, moral
panic is essentially medical panic. We have seen how medical terms
are used to embellish public discourse through references to anatomy
and physiology, to viruses, and to organs and body fluids.

Max Ricketts, a member of Pro-Life Philippines, writes "Anal sex
sabotages the immune system by the tearing of the intestinal wall and
exposure of blood and semen to fæcal matter . . ." (*Manila Bulletin*,
February 11, 1994). Ricketts' target is the homosexual. He continues:

The illusion that AIDS is essentially a sexually transmitted disease arose from
the first observations that AIDS appeared to effect only sodomites with numerous partners. However, sodomy is not sexual intercourse in the biological
sense of the words.

Homosexual men engaged in homosexual activities frequently insert their
fingers, fist, sexual organ or tongue into the lower intestinal tract of their
partners. These maneuvers transmit any virus which persists in the blood
for months or years with devastating efficiency even though no virus is present in either semen or saliva.

The sources are obviously medical texts, reread and rewritten, but the medical professionals' texts also show the social construction of "reality." Dr. Antonio Novak Feliciano and Dr. Antonio E. Feliciano Jr., a father-and-son team who claim to be experts on STDs, write in their 1990 volume of "a warning to mankind of great chastisement" from Our Lady of Fatima in 1917, "repeated by Our Lady of Akita in Japan in October 13, 1973." The Felicianos suggest that, with AIDS, "this great chastisement has started. First, with the group that made an organ for defecation into a sex organ, and now it has spread to all segments of society, including the unborn and children" (Feliciano and Feliciano, 1990, 49). Note how the Felicianos establish a vital linkage between Ricketts' sodomites infecting "all segments of society" and the health department's "general population."

There are other examples of such homophobic medical discourse (see Tan, 1994). What is more important, however, is how moral panic is created and how public discourse reflects expectations for "tools" for control—not just of HIV/AIDS but of sexuality. This control is expected from the medical world, not from drugs or vaccines, but from testing.

Much public attention has been given to the health department's epidemiological surveillance program, which receives substantial support from the United States Agency for International Development (USAID), and the choice of title itself merits analysis. USAID's current HIV program in the Philippines is in fact called the AIDS Surveillance and Education Project (ASEP). The media reports much more about the testing than about the education programs, with coverage of the latter usually limited to self-serving press releases from the more enterprising NGOs receiving funding from the project.

Officially the government opposes mandatory testing, but archaic laws require "hospitality girls" to report for testing before they can receive work permits. The women comprise one "sentinel population" (female commercial sex workers) in the surveillance program. The other "sentinel population" groups are male commercial sex workers, men who have sex with men, and injecting drug users.

Testing is described so as to assure the public the government is doing something about AIDS. A headline in *The Star*, March 17, 1992, reads "DOH Watching 50 Cities for AIDS Cases." The DOH reports on its AIDS watch using terms like "hot spot," first used in 1994 when the department disclosed that the entire Metro Manila area was a "hot spot," due to high numbers of AIDS cases. In fact, DOH had found one HIV-positive case among 302 female sex workers tested in Quezon City. Shortly after this press release, Quezon City's vice-mayor issued a press release stating that the city had created a Task Force AIDS "to arrest and contain the spread of the dreaded AIDS disease." The medical jargon is quickly internalized. In 1995, a member of the task force on AIDS in Angeles said the city should also be considered an "HIV hot spot"—dutifully defined as an area where "one out of 300 target persons is detected HIV-positive." The "hot spot" construct has been used in other ways as well. For example, during the witch hunt in Northern Samar for the two women supposedly spreading HIV, the health department told the media there was no cause for concern because Northern Samar was not a hot spot (*Today*, October 10, 1994).

The fixation over testing is complicated by the way surveillance figures are released. Quite often, there is premature release of results. Thus, when the inmates in Muntinlupa were tested, one newspaper reported: "3 Munti prisoners positive for AIDS" (*Manila Bulletin*, April 14, 1994). In reality, the test results were "indeterminate." In the end, it turned out no one tested positive, but even if the newspapers reported this clarification, it should not be surprising if the public memory retains the headline of three HIV-positive inmates.

Equally surprising are the endless attempts, at national, provincial, and municipal levels, to legislate mandatory testing. What is surprising is that health department officials, who have to testify in endless legislative sessions about the proposed mandatory testing, still have not seen the linkages between such legislative proposals and their own surveillance program. For example, some proposals are very specific in naming the groups they want to test, groups that represent a secular interpretation of the medical sentinel groups. Thus, in Cebu, there was a proposal to expand mandatory testing of women sex workers to beauticians, hairdressers, barbers, manicurists, and pedicurists because "many of them are gays who engage in homosexual activities" (*Manila Bulletin*, October 13, 1993).

Testing will remain popular for "others"—those who are supposed "at risk." And we have seen numerous examples of how testing has been used as accusation and interrogation, exculpation and acquittal, confession and judgment.

The Filipino as the "Other"

It is important to consider how AIDS impacts the ways Filipinos are seen by non-Filipinos and how moral panic relates to power relations. If some Filipinos see each visiting tourist as a possible source of HIV, there is, too, the image of tourists acquiring HIV infection in the world's favored sites for sex tourism. Note the following introduction to an article in the newsletter *World AIDS*: "A medical expert at the 1991 VIIth International AIDS conference in Italy speculated that 'every jumbo jet leaving Bangkok, Manila, Rio de Janeiro and Algiers is carrying another ten new HIV infections'" (Abbott, 1992, 5).

HIV/AIDS reconstitutes stereotypes, giving them a medical imprimatur. Instead of a single woman sex worker being a source of AIDS, we have entire nations becoming reservoirs for infection—reflecting existing power relationships, with the dominated the infectious. Liza Go, a Filipina working with overseas workers in Japan, wrote to me about receiving a card that said: "You Filipino and Thai women are the ones responsible for the spread of AIDS in Japan . . . GO HOME!!" One must remember that thousands of Filipino women are imported into Japan as sex workers; the women are "needed" but feared.

Such imagery coexists with other representations, this time of the exotic, innocent Third World native. One introduction agency, the Asia-Japan Marriage Planning Association, based in Japan, once advertised "Why don't you marry a young, healthy and beautiful Filipina and be happy? The women are office workers from healthy families and daughters of farmers. They have received medical checkups, so there is no worry of AIDS. Decide now for instant happiness!" (Cahill, 1990, 135).

These examples emphasize that the discourse reflects broader social and political contexts of sex and sexuality. It is in fact striking how legislation blatantly reflects this context. For example, Singapore requires HIV testing for its overseas workers, but only if they earn less than S$ 1500 (about US$ 1000) per month. (Singapore in fact hosts many Filipino "maids" affected by this ruling.) In the Philippines, Miriam Defensor-Santiago, while immigration commissioner, signed a circular requiring submission of "AIDS clearance certificates" for people applying for permanent visa status. Exempted from the regulations were U.S. servicemen and members of diplomatic missions, foreign aid agencies, and UN agencies. Apparently, immigration officials had forgotten another potentially powerful lobby—businessmen. In 1993, the Philippine government suspended the immigration circular for Americans, Japanese, and Europeans, after pressure from chambers of commerce.

HIV has, unfortunately, reinforced class discrimination and pooled prejudicial images: on one hand, the healthy wealthy; on the other, the diseased poor—now overlapping with images of the promiscuous. I will never forget asking, in a central Philippine city, one gay professional if we could conduct HIV prevention workshops for gay men in his area. He looked at me and said, "Not for professionals. We don't need it. We should do it for the low-class ones. They're the ones with the risky behavior." "The Other" had arrived.

The Perils of Political Correctness

One consequence of the Philippines colonial past is the rapid pace with which U.S. fads are adopted—including political correctness. Thus, journalists, politicians, and health bureaucrats have learned to use terms such as "sex workers," "men who have sex with men," and "people living with HIV." But this is often form rather than substance, and the underlying biases still emerge. Thus an article in the *Manila Times*, July 24, 1993, has a photograph captioned "A streetwalker, her head covered, undergoes AIDS tests at the Cubao police station. If found positive, her health situation will be discreetly monitored by health workers."

The article discusses how tests are conducted among "self-confessed prostitutes" in "suspected hookers' havens." Such scenes are frequently repeated, even with the cooperation of NGOs supposedly doing education and information work, complete with assurances of "voluntary testing" and "anonymity." The language is excruciatingly correct, masking the insensitivity of the activities.

There is also the use of persons with HIV as AIDS educators. Again, on the surface, this seems a very progressive policy, oriented to giving HIV a human face and providing livelihood for persons with HIV. But such a program has not been without problems. Invariably, the AIDS educators talk about how they acquired their disease from "bad behavior." Liza Enriquez, who got HIV from her Italian husband, is quoted:

I look upon my affliction as something like a punishment for my wrongdoings. I had a husband before Paolo. I left my first husband for Paolo and after that, this is what I got . . . I try to think of my disease not only as atonement for the things that I have done but I also try to see myself as an instrument of God, to make others know that AIDS attacks not only sexually active people like sex workers but also ordinary people like me.

Archie, another person with HIV used to do AIDS education, is quoted:

My sexual sojourns were so frequent that I could hardly stand a week without doing it with anybody, sometimes with women, sometimes with men. Our dilemma then was that we didn't know how to use condoms correctly.

Nick, who describes himself as bisexual, says:

By the time I was thirteen, I knew what I wanted to be. I wanted to be a girl, and started flirting with men and the funny thing was I also harbored an affection for a girl who would eventually be my wife.

The reporter writes, "Despite being married, Nick secretly bore his gender crisis until after his wife gave birth to their first child." He frequented gay bars and eventually "[fell] in love with another man." The next paragraph makes an abrupt jump: "Later on Nick began to feel the symptoms of the disease."

In effect, people with HIV end up characters in a media morality play that reinforces stereotypes. Typically, such newspaper accounts end with vacuous statements like "They now believe in the values of safe sex, which advocates abstinence from sex, fidelity to partners, and correct and consistent use of condoms in preventing the spread of the disease."

Not surprisingly, in a survey conducted by a marketing research firm (Trends/MBL, 1995), the main messages people recalled from an HIV prevention campaign were: avoid having sex with sex workers (14 percent); use Trust condoms (12 percent); avoid having sex with people you do not know (10 percent); [a neighbor complaining about having been bitten by Sarah Jane Salazar] (8 percent). Of the messages, only the first was actually found in the HIV campaign. Lay reinterpretations had apparently come in, mixing with Trust condoms' marketing and the mass media's coverage of Sarah Jane. It should be pointed out that "avoid having sex with people you do not know" grows out of popular concepts that one can "know" whether someone has HIV—certainly no effective risk-reduction measure—yet seemed to come through as a message in the campaign.

The rhetoric of political correctness runs hollow. Somehow HIV/AIDS has created channels for sanitizing, which in turn reinforce, discrimination and prejudice—sometimes with the most macabre results. I will end this section with a piece from the letters section of the *Philippine Daily Inquirer* on August 27, 1995. In 1986, Filipinos abolished the death penalty in a new constitution but a few years later brought back capital punishment for "heinous crimes." Realizing that the country's only electric chair was not working, public debates were initiated on an appropriate form of capital punishment. One Enrico Fabian writes, in opposition to proposals to use lethal injections:

If they really are looking for the most humane way to execute someone, why won't they just let the death convict have sex with a willing HIV-positive woman? The convict must not know his partner is HIV-positive, so he won't know that he's already being executed through the sexual act. That would definitely be a pleasurable death sentence. No pain, just pure pleasure.

Notice the "correct" use of terms like "HIV-positive" and "willing." Yet when the text comes together, it is clear we are witnessing an effective institutionalization of a medico-moral hegemony (Seidel, 1993).

Implications for HIV Work

I recently visited a rural health unit and remember feeling quite happy, when I entered the building, to see a bulletin board stating, in large letters, "AIDS: Shared Responsibilities." At last, I thought, even rural health units are now participating in the AIDS awareness campaigns. As I read on, however, I began to feel more distress. There were photographs showing lesions in STDs, obviously taken from African patients. On one side of the board was a picture of two women in short skirts, also wearing a cross between a smile and a smirk. And the advice on preventing HIV/AIDS included, besides the usual prescription of monogamy, abstinence, condom use, *"Iwasan ang pagpunta sa beer garden, sauna at motel"* (Avoid going to beer gardens, saunas, and motels). AIDS awareness is high in the Philippines, but this awareness is constantly shaped and reshaped by ideology and discourse. The development is not necessarily linear or progressive, and quite often campaigns that claim to inform become part of the problem. In this paper, I have described the many ways information campaigns become part of moral panic, resurrecting old—and creating new—forms of prejudice and discrimination.

One needs to understand that the medical world itself creates the conditions for this moral panic, and that the moral panic draws on a medical police model. Medical pathology becomes a base for social pathologization. The Philippines' Immigration Act of 1940, for example, bans the entry of persons with "loathsome or infectious disease," and this act was invoked in an attempt to prevent American basketball player Magic Johnson from visiting the country in 1995.

HIV/AIDS has unleashed new means of social boundary setting, for creating "the Other"—personifying the loathsome and the dreadful. Reflecting changing epidemiological patterns, "the Other" need not be the white foreigner. I have mentioned the controversy over condoms distributed to Filipino athletes heading for Thailand; newspapers reported the condom distributions were made in response "to reports that Thailand is one of the countries having the highest rate of AIDS-related cases in the world today" (*Evening Paper*, October 19, 1995).

The Other, too, can be fellow Filipinos. When a German researcher reported on camp conditions for Aeta refugees, a cultural minority group, one newspaper had the headline "Aetas May be HIV Carriers Too, Says Doc" (*Today*, October 1, 1995). A few days later, another newspaper headlined "Aetas to Undergo AIDS Test" (*Manila Bulletin*, October 5, 1995). The Aetas are Negritos and have been subject to decades of racial discrimination.

The Other is often the woman with *sakit ng babae* (women's sicknesses or STDs) spreading havoc. Tracking down such women becomes a preoccupation, especially with testing. As Sacks (1996) points out, this image—replete in the Western media as well—actually contradicts medical facts, which show that male-to-female transmission of HIV occurs more frequently than the reverse.

HIV/AIDS prevention programs become packaged as lifestyle changes, a secular version of a "moral" life. Slick campaigns are used for the social marketing of this "moral" life, with simplistic messages about abstinence and condom use—simplistic because without social context. A sex worker, for example, is presumed able to negotiate for condom use; if she cannot do so, there is always the surveillance apparatus—testing—to ensure a "cleaner" society.

The *utak pulis*—police mentality—dominates. It should not be surprising that major NGOs working in AIDS education allow themselves to be used for epidemiological surveillance, oblivious to the absurdity of voluntary testing and informed consent in bars, brothels, or even, in one instance, theaters where there was gay cruising. Not that the testing is less absurd than attempts to conduct so-called peer education and HIV training in such environments (before or after work time). Such programs betray an elitism that alternates between moralizing education—mass media messages such as "AIDS Kills" and "Don't Die of Ignorance"—and the blood-letting of testing.

The moral panic is often wrought with contradictions, for the guardians of morality are also those who would lead the country into economic recovery. Cebu City provides a good case study. Located in the central Philippines, this city is developing rapidly, with export processing zones and a tourist industry. But this development also generates AIDS-related fears. In 1992, there were proposals in Cebu to test tourists, particularly the Japanese. A news report notes, "Health Department records showed that Japan ranks third highest in Aids and HIV contamination in this part of the world, behind Australia and New Zealand" (*Manila Chronicle*, May 23, 1992). Earlier, in March of 1992, health authorities reported a rise in the number of registered sex workers in the city. The newspaper report is quite interesting in its presentation: "Apparently, the women were attracted by reports of a booming Cebu economy which had reportedly achieved a 438 percent growth in capital investments in 1988. Fresh capital amounting to U.S.$ 118 million was also reported in 1990." These business statistics are cited together with reports of "779 registered sex workers in January and February 1991 and 1557 in 1992" (*Manila Bulletin*, March 22, 1992).

Ultimately, the HIV prevention campaigns come suspiciously close to models of "social hygiene"; the term is, in fact, used for government clinics that check sex workers for STDs. One wonders if HIV prevention has not become part of the demand to keep the country clean for tourism, for business, for development, even as attempts are made to placate the guardians of morality. The new medico-moral hegemony should be recognized as not coming just from fringe conservative groups; it is reinforced through both government and private activities in HIV/AIDS prevention, often amidst secular and politically correct rhetoric. This new hegemony is all the more dangerous because often unrecognized for its subtext of surveillance, control, and stigmatization.

References

Abbott, G. (1992). "Along for the Ride: HIV and Sex Tourism." *World AIDS*, March, 5–8.

Cahill, D. (1990). *Intermarriages in International Contexts*. Quezon City: Scalabrini Migration Center.

Cohen, S. (1980 [original 1972]). *Folk Devils and Moral Panics: The Creation of the Mods and Rockers*. Oxford: Martin Robertson.

Feliciano, A. N., and Feliciano, A. E. (1990). *Sexually Transmitted Diseases*, 2d edition. Makati: Five Star Printing.

Parker, R. G. (1991). *Bodies, Pleasures, and Passions: Sexual Culture in Contemporary Brazil*. Boston: Beacon Press.

Sacks, V. (1996). "Women and AIDS: An Analysis of Media Misrepresentation." *Social Science and Medicine* 42(1):59–73.

Seidel, G. (1993). "The Competing Discourses of HIV/AIDS in Sub-Saharan Africa: Discourses of Rights and Empowerment vs. Discourses of Control and Exclusion." *Social Science and Medicine* 36(3):175–94.

Tan, M. L. (1994). "Sickness and Sin: Medical and Religious Stigmatization of Homosexuality in the Philippines." In Neil, J., Garcia, C., and Remoto, D., (eds.), *Ladlad: An Anthology of Philippine Gay Writing*, 202–19. Manila: Anvil Publishing.

Trends/MBL (1995). *Project Minuet*. KAPB Survey Commissioned by Johns Hopkins University and the Department of Health. Unpublished.

Chapter Eight

Survival Sex and HIV/AIDS in an African City

Eleanor Preston-Whyte, Christine Varga,
Herman Oosthuizen, Rachel Roberts,
and Frederick Blose

It is better to die in fifteen years' time of AIDS than to die
in five days' time of hunger.

The argument of this paper is that the context of most sex work in African cities, and probably in the countryside as well, can be summed up in a single word—survival. Shorn of controversy and emotion, sex work is about making money to remain alive, making money to feed one's children, and, in extreme cases, finding a place to "hang out" or negotiating some modicum of physical safety and protection. But it is often hard for outsiders to grasp this fact; like HIV/AIDS, sex for money or other "gifts" is an emotive issue, and both are the center of hot debates over the nature and limits of sexual relationships and acceptable sexual practice.

Bringing HIV/AIDS and sex work together highlights the elements they share in the popular imagination—multiple sex, dangerous sex, payment for sex—all activities feared to threaten social life as typified in those widespread icons of "correct" sexual life—heterosexual love, fidelity, marriage, and today of course health and survival itself. If we accept these stereotypes, and if we think of culture as a set of shared understandings that drive behavior, it is difficult to see the "culture" of sex work as mundane, pragmatic, supremely unromantic; it is easier to picture it as dangerously, excitingly, erotically illicit. Sex work may be all these things, at different times and for different people, but in most African situations, current research suggests, it is, at least from the perspective of sex workers, about surviving poverty. Sex work may indeed be dangerous, but the danger lies in the social contexts and geographical areas in which it is practiced—although there are notable exceptions, sex work tends to concentrate in the poorest and roughest parts of town. To these dangers has been added the health hazard that HIV/AIDS presents both to sex workers and to their clients. In short, sex work is about "getting by" in a world of poverty, disempowerment, and probably prejudice—a situation that applies, as we shall see, as much to male as to female sex workers.

In trying to encapsulate the above complexity, we find the term "survival sex," if not entirely original, at least useful.[1] "Survival sex" brackets sex work with other forms of small-scale informal money-making—with selling homemade items of clothing, with petty trading in fruit and vegetables, with brewing illicit liquor and running "she-beens" (local, informal, and largely illegal bars), with pick-pocketing, and with a wide range of so-called "petty crime." All over Africa, many, many women and some men, of all colors, cultures, and class backgrounds, engage in these activities at some time during their lives (Preston-Whyte and Rogerson, 1991; Bozzoli, 1991). Many combine informal money-making with formal jobs, but as unemployment grows, selling sex is, for an increasing number, the only experience of "working" to earn a living. Viewed in this light, sex is merely another commodity for sale—as using the word "commercial sex work," in preference to "prostitution," suggests so well. In the African situation, however, there are problems with the term "commercial" to cover all nuances of "sex work." Some whom the outsider might label sex workers are not always paid in hard cash; and their interaction with sex partners is relatively longlasting, with characteristics of a "relationship" rather than of a "one-off" contract for a single sexual episode. Such persons do not consider themselves prostitutes, nor do the communities in which they live and struggle to survive. Yet these persons agree they receive "gifts" and various kinds of "help" from lovers. As one woman put it, "This is how we survive."

The notion of "survival sex" emerged recently among researchers and sex workers engaged in a research project based at the University of Natal in Durban. Durban is a bustling tourist and port city on the east coast of South Africa, and we began by focusing attention on commercial sex workers servicing these aspects of city life. Initially, our research participants were drawn from the ranks of men and women who consciously depend on sex to make a living or to augment other means of survival. Most are single, although they may have long-term partners or lovers; since they have no full-time employment and seem unable to secure formal work, they look to commercial sex as their main support. They acknowledge they "sell sex" for a living, and accept the term "prostitute" to describe themselves.

A second and very different group of women have now been incorporated into our study. Some live in settled working-class communities but have few means of long-term income—except lovers who provide limited support. Others are very young women who come to Durban from nearby rural areas to buy and sell goods bought cheaply in one place and not available in another. If they have no success in selling other commodities, they may "try their luck" (in Zulu, *umuntu ophantaye*) selling sex in places known as haunts of street prostitutes. Some pass by a truck stop on the bus route home to "earn something," albeit only bus fare. They acknowledge they sell sex on these occasions, but do not regard themselves as regular long-term or "professional" sex workers. Highlighting the difference between these two categories of "sex worker" is the attitude among self-identified commercial sex workers toward men who want to treat them as "girl friends" rather than prostitutes—which would entail not necessarily receiving payment after each sexual encounter: "They [the men concerned] say they give us 'gifts' and only give money at month ends . . . We are their 'girlfriends,' so they say, and they hit us if we ask for money . . . But how do they expect us to live with no money?" Clearly, here is a blurring of categories that bears further investigation.

The above comments are from women, but male sex workers, although operating in a different milieu, tell much the same story of need; "Its really just a kind of job . . . I couldn't get another," in the words of one. It is, however, impossible to lump together all men and women who use sex for survival. Like other employment, some sex work is full-time, some part-time, some permanent, and some stop-gap. All have, however, one thing in common—and the workers recognize it—HIV/AIDS is a permanent danger, and the tragedy of their current situation is summed up in the citation that heads this chapter. The paradox of what we refer to as "survival sex," strictly commercial or not, is that relatively short-term (but nonetheless pressing) social survival is achieved only at the cost of exposure to long-term risk of illness and death.

As these introductory comments suggest, we are concerned with major social and political issues of our time—poverty, unemployment, gender disempowerment and domestic violence, sex, and the rapid spread of HIV/AIDS. Debates rage and research abounds around each topic, but there is the common theme: the use of sex to struggle for daily survival by many people in social groups that, for one reason or another, are disadvantaged and thus vulnerable. Around this theme, we build our argument and present the ethnographic work in which we are currently engaged—and out of which our argument emerged.

Sex Work and Survival in Durban

Durban is South Africa's major commercial port. It has long been a favorite holiday city for white South Africans and is an increasingly attractive international tourist destination. The city has, however, another side. Within the province of KwaZulu-Natal, Durban is a mecca for Black rural migrants in search of formal employment and of opportunities for informal money-making. Sex is one commodity, and one much in demand both among rich and poor, and it is, we argue, an integral part of the city's informal economy. Although little-remarked in the local literature, selling (and also exchanging) sex is one of the most frequent and enduring strategies used by the casual poor (see Bromley and Gerry, 1979)—and, within that category, in particular by women—to survive.

While our observations derive from work done in Durban, our conceptualization of survival sex resonates with research findings from other African cities where socially and economically disadvantaged women or men use sex as a bargaining point in relationships with those more wealthy or more powerful. The implications of our findings for understanding HIV transmission are severe, and call for urgent action with respect to intervention; if sex is, as we argue, a *survival* strategy, it is to economic and personal empowerment, as much as to education and peer counseling, that public policy must, in the long term, be directed.

Beginning to Study Sex Work in Durban

Until the advent of HIV/AIDS, little scholarly attention, with one exception (Posel and Posel, 1991), focused on commercial sex work either in Durban or in the wider KwaZulu-Natal region. Much the same was true for the country as a whole, and the "strategic silences" to which Lützen (1995) has sensitized us characterized those anthropological studies explicitly designed to deal with the behavioral intimacies and biology of sexual relationships (Varga, 1996a). It is against this background that we formed a loosely coordinated team that, working from a base provided by the University of Natal, began to explore sex work in Durban. Using a qualitative and largely anthropological approach, we aimed first to initiate an introductory ethnographic scan of commercial sex in the city and its environs. This overview was aimed at denying or confirming the diversity and complexity suggested by anecdotal evidence and reports in the popular press. This initial research resulted in a number of ethnographic vignettes of sex work in the city, which we are in process of integrating within a common analytical and theoretical framework. One of us had been, for many years, involved in studies of the informal economy of the region (Preston-Whyte and Rogerson, 1991), and this background led to the conceptual thrust of this paper, although other perspectives are emerging from our work (Varga, 1996a, 1996b).

Ethnographic Vignettes
Background

Fanning out from the harbor and beachfront, the port and inner-city holiday and tourist areas of Durban are encircled by what historically have been mostly white middle- and upper-class suburbs, parts of which are becoming multiracial. These give way to black suburbs and a sprawl of industrial and semi-industrial areas and informal settlements, which in turn shade into peri-urban, and eventually fairly dense and predominantly black rural, settlements. Public transport is slow, but it is possible from the perimeter to reach the center of this arc, or any point within it, in an hour or less by communal taxi. Holiday-makers and tourists fly in to the international airport and are transported speedily across town to the beachfront with only a glimpse of the poorer areas, where residents depend directly or indirectly on the port, beaches, and industrial sections for employment—and, as unemployment rates increase, for informal money-making opportunities. Small stalls and hawkers abound in all but the most "up-market" suburbs of the inner city, and selling sex forms part of the array of money-making strategies open both to Durbanites and to temporary migrants.

The idiom for commercial sex in Durban is predominately Western and gendered. The "trade" is said to stretch from formal "escort agencies" to "street walkers" in the "red-light district" of the so-called "Point" area, which links "dockland" and the expensive hotels of the "holiday mile." Prostitutes are conceptualized, in popular imagination and press, as *women*. Indeed, women do predominate, but there are also men who make an income in this manner. For neither these men nor most women involved is the notion of "the oldest profession" felicitous or accurate. Increasingly, commercial sex workers are black, drawn from the poorest inhabitants of the city and province—a demographic reality borne out by our fieldwork, to date concentrated on three distinct areas and social contexts in which, in Durban, commercial sex work occurs.

The first area, "the Point," includes the beachfront hotels and the traditional "red-light district" between beachfront and docks. With the exception of black domestic and service workers, this area was, as recently as five to ten years ago, the preserve of white residents and of largely white "call girls" operating from clubs, escort agencies, and flats. It is now increasingly black, in terms both of sex workers and of their clientele. In the days of apartheid, black women wishing to sell sex used dark back allies or accompanied sailors onto their ships, where local police were unlikely to challenge their activities. Such women were under constant threat of prosecution, as much for being in a "white" area and for engaging in sex across the color line as for "soliciting." Today African and Indian female (and some male) commercial sex workers frequent this area along with their white counterparts, and are becoming the majority of the sex worker population.

In the other two research areas, there are no white sex workers. The second, which we named "Industria," is a strip of mixed light-industrial and small business premises, including a small commercial hotel and a number of large truck stops. It is a rough and dangerous area, and the women working in it are tough and resilient. Most are short-term (weekly or daily) migrants from semirural areas on the Durban periphery, and engage in other income-generating strategies, such as hawking. The third research area, which we call "Suburbia," is, in contrast, a fairly typical African working-class suburb in a peri-urban area. It is in these two locations that we have explored the grey area between what the women consider "proper" commercial sex work (prostitution) and a series of longer- and shorter-term sexual relationships with men they know relatively well, for which payment is seldom in money "up front." These latter interactions have the connotation of an "exchange" rather than of a "one-off" contract. As an extension of this practice, black research participants in all three areas have complained "Our [African] men do not like to pay for sex, it is different than with whites."

Although most attention has been paid to women's sex work, one of us (Oosthuizen) worked, in the early 1990s, among men frequenting the beach area in search of clients. The rubric of sex for survival applied as much to these men as to the women in the study. A number of features, however, distinguish male from female commercial sex work in Durban, including the former's extreme fluidity, not only in personnel but in location. The "sex oasis" we shall describe has ceased to exist; both clients and sex workers have moved, and are continuously forced to move their locale of interaction. Gay sex is still controversial in some circles, and men in search of sex with other men, as well as male commercial sex workers, are far more often the focus of police attention than are their female counterparts. This point is highlighted in the following ethnography that demonstrates the marginality and insecurity of the lives of many men who sell sex to other men. At another level, commercial sex work among men is less institutionalized than between women and male clients; some also shades into non-commercial sexual exchanges.

One result of our work so far has been to raise questions about the usefulness of the blanket terms "prostitution" and "commercial sex work." Both are taken directly from non-African contexts, and neither capture the complex nuances of survival sex as we see it in Durban. In a nutshell, neither allow for the fact that "cash" may be only one of the goods for which sex is exchanged. The words of the women quoted earlier encapsulate this concern. Let us turn to our ethnography to explore such issues.

The Durban Beachfront and the Point

The Beachfront and "Point" areas are the traditional centers of commercial sex in Durban. While this is changing rapidly, it is useful to begin by describing the scene in these areas when we began fieldwork. The Beachfront is largely the preserve of "gay sex" and the haunt of male sex workers, while heterosexual sex and female sex workers dominate the "Point."

The Durban Beachfront is relatively narrow and consists of several beaches used by both locals and visitors for swimming, surfing, and sunbathing. It is separated from tourist hotels and holiday flats by a wide avenue, below which are such public facilities as an amusement park, oceanarium, snake park, eateries, and, at one point, public gardens. Changing rooms are also present, and there is a fair amount of public parking. Along this strip, two areas were at one time well-known venues for gay sex. The first was a "sex oasis," near the northern end of the beach strip, that was the accepted place to "cruise" and to which some prostitutes were attracted to service men who had not found other partners. These commercial sex workers were from all racial groups, a significant proportion African. The clients were white. This venue lost currency after a number of assaults and one killing in the near vicinity; its clientele moved to recognized bars, some in the Point area. In contrast, South Beach has long been, and continues to be, a site of regular male commercial sex trade in central Durban. It is dominated by white male prostitutes, who congregate on a large and prominent traffic island in the broad avenue above the beach area. Their number is not large; neither, however, is the demand for their services, a fact that creates competition and inclines these men to protect their "territory" from "blacks."

Male sex work is not well paid. Some of our informants claimed to make only around R 100 (U.S.$25) a night, sometimes less if they found only a single client. It is a measure of their desperation that the men remain on watch each night. Indeed, this was how informants represented themselves, and their life histories corroborate this with graphic descriptions of highly mobile and literally "homeless" people. Most had been in prison or reformatories, where they had been introduced to sex with men. Some had come to Durban from Johannesburg and the Cape, and said they would probably "move off" again once the seasonal tourist invasion of Durban was over. They had, for the most part, no fixed abode in Durban and worked "from the street." Their clients picked them up in motorcars, and sex occurred in a place usually designated by the client—often in his vehicle, on the beach, or in some other dark and deserted place. This means the sex worker was very much at the client's mercy. The following general description provides the flavor of these interactions.

Male sex workers displaying themselves on the prominent traffic island make eye contact with likely clients who drive by. They indicate to the client a convenient parking area, then go over to speak to him. The first move is to ascertain if the driver of the car is really after sex. A favorite opening line is "Looking for company?" The sex worker then initiates a discussion of terms—price and service expected. The majority of sex workers try to provide masturbation only, although they may allow themselves to be masturbated by clients. They claim they will accept anal sex only if they are the insertive partner. It is, however, difficult to get payment "up front" (that is, before the sex act), or to refuse compliance if the client is determined not to be cooperative. After the act, the sex worker is dependent on the client's willingness to return him to the beach front. Some men reported being thrown out of the car in some deserted spot and left to find their way back.

It is a lonely life that Beachfront male prostitutes live. There is little of the camaraderie of the bars and clubs of the Point area, and none of the support their women counterparts receive from colleagues. The only saving grace appears the strong likelihood that condoms will be acceptable to the clients, who are likely to be members of the local gay community. Our impression is the men we interviewed did not regard their activities as in any sense a "profession." They were "in it for the money" and would have preferred virtually any other occupation. But sex work provided an income, if a relatively small one. They were well aware of the dangers of HIV, and used condoms with most clients—indeed, it was often the clients who insisted on this. The male sex workers did not, however, carry this caution through into their own heterosexual relationships with partners.

Female sex workers were, and are, to be found not on the open beach or parking lots, but in the bars of beachfront hotels immediately behind the beach zone. Here are street upon street of mixed accommodations, from five-star international hotels to small, run-down blocks of flats. Known as "the Point"—for the headland surrounding the bay and dock area—this vicinity is often called the "red-light" district of central Durban. The Point stretches from the relatively "upmarket" beachfront to mixed-service, semi-industrial port and bay areas. In the Point are escort agencies offering massage "services" on the premises and also arranging female "escorts" for an hour or two. Interspersed between agencies are sex shops, with mildly erotic displays in their windows, and the neon-lit entrances of bars and clubs. Sex workers often stand in the doorways of these places, or hang around in the "foyers" or in front of run-down holiday hotels and blocks of flats. After about 9 A.M. or 10 A.M. the women frequent the bars opening onto the street or situated in tourist hotels.

Both the women and their clients are racially mixed. Indian and Coloured women have joined the white women who once dominated the area's commercial sex scene. The major change currently is the large number of African women moving in, as residents or as part of the "trade." Many tourists and holiday-makers are from East African countries, and these African, as well as local Indian and Coloured, clients mix with local African residents in approaching the women. A few white commercial sex workers stated that they did not accept black (African) clients, but it is clear that most women have a mixed clientele. Given the proximity to the harbor and the beachfront hotels, the clientele is also of mixed social class, language, and income. Some clients are sailors, some businessmen, and some simply male Durbanites who have frequented the area bars for years.

Apart from the sex trade, the locale is characterized by pawn shops, second-hand furniture and clothing dealers, and cheap fast-food and video stores. In the daytime, tourists as well as shopkeepers, shoppers, and prostitutes rub shoulders, and the Point is fairly safe except for the activities of ubiquitous pickpockets. At night, however, the scene changes dramatically. Neon lights flash continuously and the bars and all-night clubs come into their own. This is the haunt of a tough crowd, seeking nighttime amusement in drink, often in drugs, and in risqué floor and sex shows accompanied by loud disco music. *Dagga (cannabis)* and *mandrax* are readily available for purchase, and some sex workers use these drugs regularly; one told us she usually needed "a buzz" before going out to solicit. The relative absence of injection drug use in the area is noticeable, and makes the problems of HIV-spread less, at present, than in many other tourist and dock areas of the world. This may not, however, remain the case; police are anticipating and watching for a push toward hard drugs.

On the whole, the Point is generally threatening enough that local women prostitutes look out for each other. Many establish a base in one of the so-called "accommodation lodges," three- and four-story buildings in which rooms are rented, often by the day. In effect, these rooms are the women's homes, and they may share them with other women or with male friends. The latter do not fill the role of "traditional" pimps (in the European sense), but provide some protection for the women. If, for instance, a man's girl friend is out of the bar for longer than seems necessary, he will investigate and, if appropriate, assist her. He may also be her accomplice in "slicking clients"— that is, stealing their money.

The heterosexual sex on sale is fairly stereotypical and, on the whole, conservative. The women interviewed denied being willing to provide "kinky sex" and, in general, said they confined their services to vaginal intercourse and oral sex. Some commented that a few clients asked for anal sex, which they, for the most part, claimed to refuse; still other clients "just wanted to talk."

In this area, women sex workers operate from, and to some extent move between, escort agencies, massage parlors, bars, clubs, and the street. While the escort and massage services offered by agencies and parlors are legal, sex acts with clients are illegal. Many older female sex workers who have been working and living in the area for some years have been arrested, prosecuted, and fined. They are known to the police and, indeed, know the local police just as well. They are reputedly subject to some violence and even sexual exploitation at the hands of police, but, on the other hand, can rely on the police to attempt to assist and protect them when necessary. Suspected drug offences are often the cause of police harassment, although "slicking" also can bring prosecution.

Compared with the situation in the other areas studied, commercial sex work in the Point is predictable and well organized, and newcomers are soon integrated into "the system." What can only be described as a "contract" is negotiated before a woman goes with a client or invites him to her room. Although the black women are not all proficient in English or Afrikaans, they know enough to state their fee, and are supported in this by colleagues. Payment must be made before sex takes place, and, for their own safety, women prefer that sex occur in their rooms. This allows male friends or other women to gauge how long has elapsed and to investigate if necessary. In cases where women accompany men in their cars, their fellows take the registration number. Some women who operate on the streets have established territories, over which disputes may arise should another move in. More often, personal animosities flare up, especially when the individuals have been drinking heavily.

Significant differences occur in age and experience between the white prostitutes and their African counterparts. The former are older; many interviewed were in their late twenties and thirties, very few under twenty. None of the white women we interviewed were new to prostitution or to the Point; they knew their clientele and were "streetwise" and "at home." In contrast, many of the black women were very young, and some had been working in the Point area for only a month or so. In the bars, the younger and less experienced women tended to cluster around the dance floors, actively seeking to attract clients, while the older women sat at the bar counters. Some of the latter had regular customers—in time, most women would come to operate from particular bars. The population of prostitutes in the bars and on the streets changed fairly rapidly, and there was room for considerable individuality. A feature of white prostitutes in the area was their language background; all were Afrikaans-speaking, and although they might speak English with clients, Afrikaans was the primary language of interaction between them and their personal partners. (Much the same may be said of male sex workers on South Beach.) The African women spoke either Zulu or Xhosa as their home language, but had some knowledge of English—less frequently, of Afrikaans, although most communication with clients was conducted in the latter. Most of the African' women had completed four or more years of school; and in keeping with white educational norms, most of the white women had three or four more years' schooling.

Over time, we have been struck by the rapid changes in the demographic composition of the women operating in the Point area. The life histories we have collected show strikingly that both white and black women are themselves highly mobile. The former take off to visit other towns; the latter move in and out of commercial sex work. Some white women claimed to be seeking other jobs. What often draws women back is the relatively high income possible from commercial sex work in the Point. A reasonable average is between R 100 and R 300 per night (U.S.$25–75), for either a white or a black woman.

In the Point, one dimension of "formality" is the general acceptance of condom use by both commercial sex workers and clients. The women openly discuss AIDS and STDs, and most stated they would not accept a client who would not wear a condom. In more intimate discussions, the temptation was acknowledged to let this rule slip for "big money," but most women pointed out that the majority of white clients were as insistent as they on "safe sex." Where the women were most vulnerable was in being unaware that particular lubricants could cause the condom to split. Those women reporting cases of condom splitting seemed fairly fatalistic about it. None were using condoms with their partners, and some acknowledged that, with long-standing clients, too, they "sometimes forgot"; the almost universal tendency of sex workers to separate professional and private lives was only too apparent in the Point area. In addition, while most of these women had had an STD, they had received treatment; there is easy access to hospital and clinic treatment for all area residents, and women were heard encouraging friends to use these facilities.

The general impression is that commercial sex workers in the Point are reasonably satisfied with their lives. Sex work there pays well, and the black women in particular appreciate that the money and social environment are far better than in other areas of Durban. Indeed, some have migrated from areas like Industria or very like Suburbia. The contrast between the Point and the latter areas could hardly be more stark.

All the women interviewed were open about their "job." They acknowledged being sex workers, and the white women described themselves as "prostitutes" with no apparent hesitation. African women referred to each other as *"isipunta,"* a local word for "prostitute." At one time, a woman who had worked in the Point for many years attempted to start a union. This was reported in the press and on television, and although it faded fairly soon, it is remembered by both sex workers and their "clients," in the bars, and is given as an example of the camaraderie and, perhaps, "respectability" of sex work in the area. Certainly, long-term clients and bar and hotel owners and managers agree that prostitutes are part of the economic life of the Point. They acknowledge the women bring people to the area and are even a tourist attraction.

While in the above respects female sex workers in the Point area form a single category, there is little doubt they are divided by racial history. The black women are relative newcomers—at least, only fairly recently have they been accepted in the bars and clubs in large numbers. Not only are most younger than the majority of the white women, they experience problems their white counterparts do not. All commented that black (African) clients were often loath to pay for sex, a tendency that presented difficulties and sometimes led to fights. This theme runs, in fact, through all our data on black hetero-sexual sex work in Durban.

Industria

Situated some six kilometers from the center of Durban and from the Point, Industria is part of Durban's urban sprawl. It was formerly an Indian residential area, but its population has become mixed as Africans have settled or rented rooms in the suburb to be close to the city and to the abutting light industrial and factory areas. Starting as a "strip" development along a large main road leading out of Durban, Industria has become a mixed residential and business area. Family businesses exist side-by-side with small factories and shops, and many residents live above or behind their establishments. There are tearooms selling food items and refreshments and keeping long business hours, a few "nightclubs," and at least one seedy hotel, outside which female sex workers congregate to attract clients and to pass the time. Relatively few of these women live in the area. Here, in contrast to the Point, sex is mostly sold by African women who live in adjacent suburbs or travel into Industria from nearby shack settlements—or even more distant rural areas. The majority are very young, but know a visit to Industria is a way to make some cash. The women soon become streetwise but, in the process, they experience harassment and violence both from clients and from the area's ubiquitous gangs.

Industria is rough and poverty-stricken; it has a high crime rate and little police presence or protection. The gangs roaming the streets impose their will on residents and transients alike. There are at least three large truck depots, and the presence of many truck drivers passing through attracts commercial sex workers. Some women enter into long- or short-term relationships with truckers; this may entail not only arranging to be available when the trucker visits Durban, but, on occasion, traveling with him in the cab of his truck. This gives some sex workers opportunity to visit other truck stops, even to work briefly in other parts of the country.

In addition to the truckers' ready call on their services, prostitutes have good and fairly regular opportunities for "one-off" commercial sex encounters with Indian and African men living in, or on the fringes of, the area or coming there in search of sex. The chance for these encounters, as much as anything else, attracts women to Industria and keeps them working there despite the dangers. A number of women described being forced to undergo an "initiation" when they began working there; this consisted of being raped by one or more local toughs (*tsotsis*) who "patrol" the local streets. All in all, Industria is an unpleasant and dangerous environment, particularly for women, and it is a measure of their desperation that the female sex workers we interviewed work there. In a real sense, they are at equal or greater risk of abuse from local criminal elements than from clients.

Given this setting, the conditions under which the women offer sex in Industria are bad. Since many have no base in the area, they have little protection from clients, from criminals, from the elements, or from extremes of climate. When approached for sex, they have no alternative but to enter a client's vehicle, after which they have no protection from abuse and no means of enforcement if the client refuses to pay. Moreover, few women manage to negotiate any sort of understanding on payment or kind of service expected, before entering the client's car—and, in so doing, his power. Industria sex workers reported far higher levels of abuse (rape, robbery, and general violence) from clients than did women working at the Point.

The women are vulnerable too, because commercial sex is much less organized and formalized than in the Point area, and they do not have the protection of male partners living with them. Many begin sex work out of desperation when, having traveled to Durban as itinerant traders and found no market for their goods, they are forced to find some way to make money. Many, despite their youth, are providing the main income for a family. Those who live relatively close to Durban travel to Industria each afternoon and return home late at night or in the early morning.

On the whole, this is a highly mobile sex-worker community, with individuals appearing and disappearing as need drives them. There are similar areas nearby where sex work is readily available, and, if unsuccessful in Industria, the women move off to try their luck elsewhere. Most are thus essentially street prostitutes, although a relatively small, slightly more stable group of women work out of the small local hotel and two nightclubs in the area. Most of the women have a good deal of experience in walking the streets, usually in threes and fours for protection and, to some degree, for company; beyond this, there is seldom much mutual support. After some time working the area, most women explore the truck stops, and some establish long-term relationships with one or a series of truckers; their place in the open streets is taken by new and younger recruits from the country or the shack regions.

In general, life at the truck stops is less hard than on the streets. The truckers are often tired and make few demands beyond rapid sex. Some "just want company" and allow the women to rest and even sleep in the cabs of their vehicles. Few drink to excess, as they must not drive under the influence of liquor, so fights are at a minimum. In comparison with the street scene, the truck depot is almost orderly. Once women establish longer relationships with truckers, they have protectors—unless the visits of two "boyfriends" coincide. Even then, the men usually appear understanding of the nature of the prostitute's life.

As at the Point, the women working in Industria see themselves as commercial sex workers, but it is important that they do not view prostitution as their primary "profession." Even the older women and those working from the hotel and bars say they have been temporarily forced into sex work and wish to leave it eventually. For most, it is only one of a wide range of small-scale money-making strategies for survival. The young traders from the rural areas most exemplify this combination of sex work and selling goods, but most of the women at some point had goods for sale, and the truckers often brought goods acquired on their travels for their "girl friends" to sell.

Few women we interviewed are heavy drinkers or smokers, and even those working from the hotel and bars are far less sophisticated than their counterparts in the Point. Because so many are young and inexperienced, they have difficulty negotiating—let alone enforcing— any agreement they may manage to make with a client. Part of their naiveté comes from low educational achievement. None matriculated, and the average claim school attendance only through sixth or seventh standard. This also limits their ability to obtain formal employment and makes them dependent on itinerant money-making strategies. Their rural background, too, often renders them naive, at least at first, and financially desperate. Since many work to support extended families at home, they cannot return empty-handed. They often accept very low payments; the young girls from shack areas near Industria sometimes give sex for the equivalent of "bus fare home," particularly late at night and in the early morning. Although most would like, they say, to insist on condom use, realistically they cannot negotiate this, and may have to accept as little as R 20 (U.S.$5) for their services, and this invariably means without a condom. On a "good day," these street prostitutes net about R 125 (U.S.$25) for a night's work; usually their total is less.

One aspect of sex work in Industria needs further comment; a woman who gravitates to the truck depots often develops, with a particular man, an ongoing relationship of a fairly complex and subtle nature. While she will solicit other clients, such a sex worker will, as noted previously, make herself available for the trucker when he is in Durban. In some cases he does not pay after each exchange of sex; instead, he provides a monthly allowance and sometimes also buys clothes, food, and soap for her. Sometimes she only receives "gifts," blurring the nature of the contractual relationship with the trucker; he is both client and personal partner, or "boyfriend." Several truckers reported "falling in love" with a beautiful young sex worker at the depot and deciding to seek her company whenever in Durban. When a relationship of this sort develops, it can prove problematic, as the man, soon feeling he does not have to pay for sex each time, may give the woman relatively small "gifts" but claim that he is supporting her by giving money "each month." She may then begin to feel "out of pocket," and complain, "black men won't pay . . . they just want us to be their sweethearts." The trucker may feel, however, that he has established a different sort of relationship than he would have with a prostitute—his gifts are "just to please the girl," not to pay her as a "street woman." (Here, the relationship of Industria women with truckers merges with the type of protective relationship observed in the area we call "Suburbia.") It is also possible—probable—that women who develop these relationships with truckers may be replicating relationships with lovers at home. In such cases, it becomes difficult to speak of "commercial sex" in the Western sense, and the term "survival sex" becomes appropriate.

As noted, most women working on the streets in Industria reported that the black men they serviced did not want to pay for sex from black women. This attitude can easily lead to fights and violence against sex workers demanding to be paid. It is our impression that many younger women working in Industria accept this situation, or are too naive and afraid to insist on payment; operating in lonely areas away from the open streets, they seldom have support, and prefer to escape open violence rather than press a claim. This links to inability to insist on—even, in most cases, to suggest—the use of condoms. Most of the women, however, are well aware of the possible dangers of HIV/AIDS; they discussed this openly with us, some recounting how sex workers they had known had died of AIDS. Their general attitude was one of fatalism. AIDS is seen as a "job hazard" but, as one woman said, "What can we do?" And where a trucker is becoming a "boyfriend," there is less possibility than ever of insisting on a condom. All the women interviewed reacted negatively to the suggestion of using condoms with "boyfriends" or husbands, and trucker "boyfriends" were said to be especially uncomfortable about condom use.

Although young and mostly single, all the women already had, or expected to have, lovers at home. Thus they were, and are, providing a continuously changing sexual link between urban Durban, the shack settlements, and the rural areas. With truckers (and some sex-worker partners) moving continuously through rural areas to conurbations north, south, and west of Durban, the network of potential HIV infection spreads and grows ever denser.

Suburbia

In contrast to the Point and Industria, "Suburbia" was established as an African area and has remained effectively uniracial. It is situated about fifteen kilometers from Durban and was built in the early 1960s as a formal "township" to house Africans and so keep them to the outskirts of the white apartheid city. Today, Suburbia forms part of a populous conurbation totaling approximately 45,000 persons, and has the general character of a settled, if poor and predominantly working-class, suburb.

Suburbia was designed on a typical "township" plan, with sites set aside for three schools (estimated sufficient to serve its targeted population), community center, small business center, light-industrial complex, two primary-health clinics, and a migrant workers hostel. The latter, still operational, reputably provides a focus for what we term informal sex work; we have not yet investigated this, but some of our research participants say they went to the hostel to "meet men."

Our work in Suburbia has concentrated on how local women between roughly the ages of eighteen and thirty use sex to survive—in a very particular way. By and large, the women are single, have one or more small children, and live with parents or other kin in the suburb. They need more financial support than their parents are able or willing to provide but have little hope of finding a job. They also want a "good time," which they seek through having a number of lovers. Their relationships with men are best described as "exchange relationships" and, if we would use the term "sex worker," we must term them "informal sex workers." The exchange relationships may be short- or long-term, and revolve around the man's provision of some material security in return for sexual relations. Material support ranges from food, clothing, shelter (usually fairly temporary, the women generally living with their extended kin and with their children, if any), money, and limited, temporary physical protection.

The women are pragmatic about their motives. One commented, "We live this way in order to survive"; another explained that she, like many others, fostered several exchange relationships simultaneously; and still another claimed that up to six such relationships at a time was not unusual for her. The women spend a few nights with a man, then "mysteriously" disappear to the next. They list their expectations as "money, clothes, soap, and so on." However, any reference or question as to the amount or regularity of this is not welcomed; similarly, any suggestion that there is a direct trade of sex for cash is denied— and usually brings the interview to an abrupt close. These women deny being prostitutes and do not see themselves in the same light as they see women sex workers of the Point or Industria. It is important that, while women we interviewed in both other areas saw themselves as sex workers, Suburbia women did not for a moment so categorize themselves—nor did the men with whom they had relationships or, for that matter, the community at large. However, few women had formed long-standing relationships with their men, but seemed to move easily from one to another.

The Suburbia women we interviewed have not yet reached the point in their lives of needing to be concerned about "settling down" or establishing their own homes. This will come when their parents and older kin begin to age and die, leaving fewer and fewer homes where they can find shelter for their growing children. At such time, they may seriously think about additional ways to earn money. With an education through the sixth standard or so, they are likely to be limited to domestic work—poorly paid and unpopular—trading, or running shack shops and shebeens. Surviving will then take on a new and more serious meaning, and may dictate a different sexual strategy. Which women are drawn into full commercial sex work, and which follow other routes to survive, needs further investigation.

What are the downsides of the "exchange" type of relationship and life? First, the woman is at the sole mercy of the man or men with whom she has relationships. They meet on the man's terms and in his (or a friend's) room. Signs of physical violence such as bruises and cuts are often present, and having a number of lovers at once clearly risks jealousy and misunderstanding. There is, of course, no formal contract, not even a formal verbal agreement, between the parties. The relationship begins and takes its course with the man essentially in the more powerful position. Some of the women drink and smoke fairly heavily, and so do their men. If the women frequent shebeens to meet men, they may become embroiled in fights. Some women seek attachments with local taxi drivers, and this is currently a dangerous occupation, due to taxi feuds. The women choose men who appear prosperous, but these men often believe their wealth confers exclusive rights. Since the men may also cultivate many women friends, the "girl friends" may eventually come to blows.

However, the real danger for these Suburbia women lies in that they rarely, if ever, use condoms. In fact, discussion of condoms in Suburbia has proved very difficult and sensitive. As in much of the general black community, condoms are associated with promiscuity, disease, and uncleanness. Most women in Suburbia are loath to be associated with condoms; they say that, if found in possession of a condom, they will be branded "disease-ridden whores." The very notion of using a condom with a husband or lover, or in an exchange relationship, is unthinkable. It would, the women say, jeopardize the relationship. In any case, they argue, they cannot set the terms of the sex act and, if they try, will be branded a "prostitute." The prevalence of such notions gives cause for grave concern, the more so as associations of condoms and condom use with being "dirty" or having "diseases such as AIDS" appears a developing social construction. As the HIV epidemic spreads and is publicized, the beliefs and fears associated with it grow, concretize, become entrenched. What we are being told in Suburbia is an important indicator of this process. It is ironic that this particular construction should turn on notions of sex for "commercial" purposes—the very concept not seen as a component of the nonmarital sexual relationships prevalent in Suburbia.

To give point to the above, most women we have been working with in Suburbia have never used a condom. Although they, like women in the other areas studied, are relatively well informed about STDs and HIV/AIDS, and do believe that HIV/AIDS exists, they are essentially fatalistic. Their attitude is that they have other pressing problems to consider; hence our initial quotation, from a Suburbia woman, "It's better to die in fifteen years' time of AIDS than to die in five days' time of hunger."

Survival Sex and the Informal Sector

The Suburbia woman's words have an all-too-familiar ring for any researcher steeped in the literature and experience of the "informal sector" in Durban. Leaving aside the specific reference to AIDS, much the same remarks are made by men and women engaged in many of the dangerous and illegal forms of informal money-making that abound in the city's poorer areas. Perhaps the closest and most apt parallel is found in descriptions of the early years of city history, when African women brewed beer and other illegal liquor for sale to the growing community of migrant men in the single-sex hostels and the shack areas surrounding the port and the growing town. The she-beens where the various brews were sold were places of social conviviality, and sex soon became an additional attraction. Durban was not unique. One of the earliest descriptions of women's involvement in informal money-making in South Africa comes from a paper on "beer brewing" in the Cape (Hunter, 1993); Hellmann's (1948) classic description of a "slum yard" in Johannesburg echoes the same points. In Durban, women still recall the days when their stills were regularly raided by municipal police and they had not only to pay fines but to begin their business anew. In field-notes made nearly twenty-five years ago, this quotation catches the spirit of the time: "It happens the police know we brew to live, but they have to chase us . . . We just pay the fines and begin again, and then they have to come again . . . but what can we do? . . . We have to take a chance . . . We women have no other jobs, and the money the men get is so small it can't feed our children." The *ongoing* structural relationship of poverty and risk is clear; all that has changed is that HIV has made the "chance" women take a matter not only of survival, but of death.

The brewer's remarks highlight a number of other important points.

For women with no or little education, there is very limited formal
employment available. Even for the present generation, for whom
education is relatively more common, jobs are hard to find. But, as
elsewhere in the world, women's domestic skills—including sex—are
in demand where men migrate and live in hostels or shacks. Making
and selling food, selling fruit and vegetables, selling small items of
cheap clothing—all complement selling liquor. Other authors have
commented that women in the informal sector simply extend their
existing capabilities—stereotyped generally as women's work—to
serve the needs of their fellows but are seldom paid well for the effort
(Moser, 1984). Writers on the informal economy often distinguish
between businesses that generate enough profit to plough back into
expanding the operation and those in which only enough is made to
assist basic survival (Dewar and Watson, 1981). By far the majority of
women working in the informal sector fall into the latter category,
and their participation in the informal economy is characterized by
low returns for long hours and poor working conditions. Although
"shebeen queens" are romanticized in the popular imagination as
larger (and more beautiful) than life, and are rumored to "make a
packet," success stories are the exception (Edwards, 1988). Most liquor sellers, like other informal sector operators, exist, if not literally
at a "survivalist" level, at least near it. Our data suggests this is also
the case with sex workers. There may be women who service wealthy
men and consortia, working out of exclusive nightspots, but they are
not the run-of-the-mill women working in escort agencies or frequenting the seedy bars and back streets of Durban. It is the latter
who are in the majority and whose work we liken to other, often highly
exploitative, forms of informal sector money-making engaged in from
necessity rather than choice. Theirs are the "desperation" strategies.
(See, on such strategies in other contexts, Cross and Preston-Whyte,
1983.)

Conclusions: Survival Sex and HIV/AIDS in Durban

In concluding, let us review what our research has so far revealed
about the field of "survival sex" in Durban. First, this terrain is broad;
it stretches from what is clearly perceived and accepted by prostitutes
and most clients as "commercial sex work" in the usual Western sense
to, at the far extreme, a much more informal and essentially ambig-

uous category of action for which the term "commercial" is not appropriate, and for which such a description is, certainly, contested by the "actors." These poles are represented concretely in our ethnographies, but they could be seen as ideal types set along an arc, with the Beachfront and Suburbia forming the two extremes. Between, Industria stands, a point in what may be a complex gradation of situations and contexts. In Industria we also encounter, in the case of truckers, a situation in which sex workers and clients interpret the nature of their interaction differently; while the women seek to be paid for services, as might any commercial sex worker, the men see the interaction as a "relationship" closer to that prevailing in Suburbia.

Indeed, since Durban is still made up of relatively discrete suburbs based on race, it is likely that further exploration will find other, possibly even more complex, sex "arenas," including some exploited by Indian, Coloured, and white women—and men. Class and language may be contextual variables and pointers, as may education and differential employment opportunities, as well as opportunities for informal money-making. Our model, however, is almost infinitely extendible, of use for a variety of descriptive or analytical purposes (Varga, 1996a).

Second, while the nodes in the social field are likely, at one level, to be characterized by fairly discrete and dense social networks, the evidence so far is that some individuals move between and among the nodes, at least over time. In doing so, they carry their sexual histories with them—and if they are HIV-infected, render their new clients and personal partners vulnerable. We need to get a handle on the magnitude of this movement very soon; as yet, our work has been purely qualitative and exploratory.

Third, the simple model we have developed, we believe, allows us not only to visualize the social field but to target particular nodes or areas for appropriate intervention. Because of its simplicity, this model will, we believe, appeal to policy and decision makers in the health field. In South Africa, the notion of "sexual networks" has already entered the discourse of health professionals in the HIV/AIDS field, although it has yet to be either fully understood or operationalized in research or intervention.

Fourth, on issues of race and gender, our model allows us to map the influence of, and—critically, in the fast-changing present political milieu—the changes in, these arenas. This information, and especially public awareness of it, is critical at a time a new constitution is under negotiation. Cultural assumptions about sexual behavior and HIV need to be opened for debate; traditional stereotypes and "silences" must be confronted. And it is here that good research can help—both to demystify and to end those silences, at present probably life-threatening for much of the population in general, and for women in particular. Sex workers, as our research clearly shows, are vulnerable even if they use condoms with clients, since they do not carry this protection into sexual relations with personal partners; vulnerability is greater still among those women who do not perceive themselves as sex workers and who cannot negotiate condom use with potentially numerous partners. And any research findings that indicate resistance to condom use, and especially those that point to the development of negative associations, as is clearly occurring in Suburbia, must be speedily fed into intervention programs.

Using the brief and selective ethnographies presented above, we can begin to compare areas and nodes, within the total social field of sex work in Durban, in terms of characteristic "risk factors." Our ethnographies, for instance, immediately present stark area-wide differences in condom use with clients and in the associated ability of women sex workers to negotiate a "contract" including condom use. The amount netted from individual clients for a particular period of time (usually conceptualized by "the night") is also rendered comparable, and reflects the need ("desperation," in some areas) of the women (and men) concerned. The features of the social background producing this vulnerability can then be mapped, providing indications of possible areas for support and intervention.

We suggest, finally—and strongly—that successful intervention in the HIV/AIDS field will need a broad-based approach not only targeting the HIV and health arenas, but developing strategies to remove such structural barriers to survival as inability to find alternative income sources. In the literature on HIV intervention, much is made of the need to empower people, women in particular, to take control of their own lives and sexual decisions. Academic education and economic self-sufficiency go together, and would seem critical in this. If we accept the notion that sex work is but one part of the informal sector—allied, furthermore, to the poorest, most exploited part of this sector—we must acknowledge the extreme vulnerability of its participants, a vulnerability that can only be ameliorated as those concerned are able to find employment sufficiently well paid; alternatively, their informal money-making activities must transcend the survivalist or desperation level. Only in such a way will they be able to move out of sex work and the survivalist section of the informal economy.

Notes

1. "Survival sex" is a term coined, in a related context, by Muir (1991).

References

Bozzoli, B. (1991). "The Meaning of Informal Work: Some Women's Stories." In Preston-Whyte, E. M., and Rogerson, C., (eds.), *South Africa's Informal Economy*, 15–33, Cape Town: Oxford University Press.

Bromley, R., and Gerry, C. (eds.). (1979). *Casual Work and Poverty in Third World Cities*. Chichester: John Wiley.

Cross, C., and Preston-Whyte, E. M. (1983). "The Informal Sector: Desperation versus Maximisation Strategies." *Indicator South Africa*, 1(2):9–12.

Dewar, D., and Watson, V. (1981). "Urban Planning and the Informal Sector." In Preston-Whyte, E. M., and Rogerson, C., (eds.), *South Africa's Informal Economy*, 181–95, Cape Town: Oxford University Press.

Edwards, I. (1988). "Shebeen Queens: Illicit Liquor and the Social Structure of Drinking Dens in Cato Manor." *Agenda*, 3:75–97.

Hellmann, E. (1948). *Rooiyard: A Sociological Survey of an Urban Native Slum Yard*. Cape Town: Oxford University Press.

Hunter, D. J. (1993). "AIDS in Sub-Saharan Africa: The Epidemiology of Heterosexual Transmission and the Prospects for Prevention." *Epidemiology*, 4(1):63–72.

Lützen, K. (1995). "La mise en discours and Silences in Research on the History of Sexuality." In Parker, R. G., and Gagnon, J. H., (eds.), *Conceiving Sexuality: Approaches to Sex Research in a Postmodern World*, 19–31, New York and London: Routledge.

Moser, C. O. N. (1984). "The Informal Sector Reworked: Viability and Vulnerability in Urban Development." *Regional Development Dialogue*, 5(2): 135–78.

Muir, M. (1991). *The Environmental Context of AIDS*. New York: Praeger.

Posel, R., and Posel, D. (1991). "Women and Gender in Southern Africa." Paper presented at the Conference on Women and Gender in Southern Africa. University of Natal, Durban.

Preston-Whyte, E. M., and Rogerson, C. (eds.). (1991). *South Africa's Informal Economy*. Cape Town: Oxford University Press.

Varga, C. (1996a). "The Commercial Sex Industry in Durban, South Africa:

A Conceptual Life History of a Sex Worker (Working Results)." Paper presented at the Joint Conference of the Pan African Anthropological Association and the Association for Anthropology in Southern Africa. UNISA, Pretoria, 2–13 September.

————. (1996b). "The Symbolism and Dynamics of Condom Use among Commercial Sex Workers in Durban, South Africa." Paper presented at the Joint Conference of the Pan African Anthropological Association and the Association for Anthropology in Southern Africa. UNISA, Pretoria, 2–13 September.

Chapter Nine

Cultural Regulation, Self-Regulation, and Sexuality

A Psycho-Cultural Model of HIV Risk in Latino Gay Men

Rafael M. Diaz

Quantitative studies of Latino gay/bisexual men in the U.S. have revealed a positive, statistically significant correlation between individuals' intentions to practice safer sex and their reported condom use in sexual encounters (Diaz, 1995). The correlation suggests, as expected, that individuals who consistently use protection tend to report stronger intentions and commitments to practice safer sex than do individuals who engage in sexual risk behavior. Yet, although the relationship is statistically significant, stated intention to practice safer sex is only a weak predictor of safer sex behavior in this population, explaining only about 3 percent of the variance in reported condom use. A substantial number of study participants who had not protected themselves also reported personal plans, strong intentions, and explicit commitments to use condoms for HIV prevention. The finding that a relatively strong personal intention to practice safer sex may coexist with the practice of unprotected or unsafe sexual behavior is not only psychologically puzzling but in need of further explanation.

Crucial to the task of HIV prevention is to understand the variables, factors, and contexts that compete with enactment of personal intentions of safer sex. Even with relatively strong intentions, an individual may encounter situations that undermine their enactment. Our task is to understand the nature of such situations, as well as the processes and mechanisms by which individuals may, or may not, overcome the obstacles to safer sex practices. Those obstacles or barriers might be personal (psychological or subjective), contextual (cultural, social, interpersonal), or both (psycho-cultural)—as when cultural guidelines become cognitive scripts that guide sexual behavior. Repeated failure to enact personal intentions may lead to a sense of helplessness and fatalism that threatens perceived self-efficacy and weakens the formulation and enactment of future intentions (Bandura, 1994). If "weakened" intentions are indeed a significant predictor of unsafe sexual practices, then we must understand the factors causing such weakening.

A major goal of the present paper is to document the search for person–situation variables that disrupt enactment of behavioral intentions in the domain of safer sex among Latino gay/bisexual men in the U.S. This search has paved the way for a psycho-cultural theoretical framework or model to help us understand how sociocultural factors shape and regulate sexual activity in this group, at times competing against self-regulatory enactment of safer sex intentions. The theoretical framework thus attempts to model the dynamic tension between cultural regulation and self-regulation in the practice of safer sex. The label "psycho-cultural" underscores the socialization/developmental viewpoint that cultural guidelines and sociocultural factors are not simply part of environmental context, not merely external to individuals. Rather, the model assumes that cultural guidelines become intrapsychic, internalized cognitive scripts and learned emotional responses that become major psychological regulators of sexual behavior.

The psycho-cultural model of HIV-risk addresses the possibility that, in the face of strong personal and interpersonal pressures against condom use, or of competing factors, there might be a breakdown of intentional/volitional processes in the sexual activity of Latino gay men. In other words, the model suggests that, faced with strong competing factors, intentions may not simply be replaced by new or different intentions; rather, the psychological organization of intentional activity may collapse in favor of more automatized, routine habitual functioning independent of personal behavioral intent. I use the term "volitional breakdown" to refer to this hypothesized collapse of intentional activity.

The model proposes, moreover, that, in the face of volition breakdown, cultural guidelines internalized as cognitive scripts, rather than personally formulated intentions, become the main regulators of sexual activity. Thus, the proposed model attempts to integrate two seemingly contradictory propositions—namely, that culture is a major regulator of human sexuality (Gagnon and Simon, 1973; Parker, 1991), and that many individuals are able to exercise considerable self-direction and self-regulation (Bandura, 1994) in the domain of sexual behavior. Such an integrative explanation is needed because, as will be shown, data on Latino gay/bisexual men reveal both self-regulatory strength and cultural disruptions of volitional control in the practice of safer sex.

For two important reasons, an explanation of intention–behavior inconsistencies is particularly pressing for the field of HIV prevention research. First, many theories of behavioral change in the field have focused on the processes by which individuals come to formulate behavioral intentions, rather than on the processes or circumstances through which the intentions can, or cannot, be enacted. Second, there is substantial evidence that a number of interpersonal variables (for example, peer pressure, sexual coercion, threat of rejection), as well as personal variables (decreased pleasure, sexual discomfort, pressing needs for intimate contact and connection), compete rather strongly with the enactment of well-meaning safer sex intentions formulated by sexually active, presumptively at-risk, individuals.

This paper has four major sections. The first presents a critique of current models of behavior change, especially those Western psychological and health models that assume individual cognitive/volitional control over sexual behavior. The second, based on qualitative data on Latino gay men, describes sociocultural factors that regulate the men's sexual behavior and that may explain discrepancies between their personal intentions and actual behavior. The third section explores constructs of culture and self-regulation as a conceptual foundation for a new model of HIV risk in Latino gay men. Finally, the fourth section proposes an outline for a psycho-cultural model of sexual self-regulation that dynamically integrates the impact of culture and self-regulation in the practice of safer sex.

Even though this psycho-cultural model of risk is being developed in the context of data from Latino gay/bisexual men in the U.S., it is my belief that the model can be adapted and applied to any group or individuals exhibiting discrepancies between personal intentions and actual behavior.

Models of Behavior Change
for HIV Prevention

The overwhelming majority of HIV prevention research in the U.S. has been guided by a limited set of relatively well known "models of behavior change": the Health Belief Model; the Theory of Reasoned Action; the AIDS Risk Reduction Model (ARRM); Prochaska and DiClemente's Stages of Change Model; Bandura's Social Cognitive Theory; and, more recently, Fisher and Fisher's Information–Motivation–Skills (I-M-S) Model of HIV Risk Behavior. These models have been useful and productive on many counts. For example, perceived self-efficacy, as postulated by Bandura, has emerged as a significant predictor of sexual risk behavior in most studies that measured the variable (Coates et al., 1988). Similarly, recent analyses by Fisher et al. (1994) have documented their model's ability to predict about 28 percent of the variance in sexual risk behavior reported by samples of (mostly white) American college students.

As theoretical guides for HIV prevention research and interventions, however, the majority of these models are seriously limited:

1.   With the exception of the ARRM and I-M-S, the models were originally formulated for domains other than sexuality and drug use, and in contexts other than HIV prevention;

2.   the models typically emphasize, and/or were designed to predict, the personal formulation of individuals' behavioral intentions;

3.   even though many of the models give some weight to the impact of social norms on individuals' behavior, each assumes that the behavior in question is under individual volitional control. In other words, the models assume that if individuals' intentions are strong enough, behavior will follow.

In an integrating "Theorist's Workshop" sponsored by the National Institute of Mental Health (Fishbein et al., 1991), a group of influential American theorists explored points of both convergence and debate, in efforts to understand behavior prediction and behavior change in the context of HIV prevention. Early in the workshop's report, these theorists underscored two major points of consensus or agreement.

The first was that AIDS transmission is a consequence of an individual's behavior: "AIDS is first and foremost a consequence of behavior. It is not who you are, but what you do that determines whether or not you expose yourself to HIV, the virus that causes AIDS" (Fishbein et al., 1991, 1).

While justly attempting to move away from biased notions relating HIV transmission to membership in "risk groups," the theorists went to another extreme; by locating the causes of HIV transmission in individual behavior, they moved away from structural or cultural analysis of human behavior, where sexual behavior can be understood as regulated by sociocultural, political, and economic structures, especially the power structures shaping and determining gender-appropriate norms and behavior (see for example Amaro, 1995). Interestingly, the theorists defined AIDS transmission in the context of individual behavior even though clear epidemiological data in the U.S. located the virus not in random distribution across the population but in specific contexts defined by social experiences of poverty, racism, and homophobia within minority populations (National Commission on AIDS, 1992). It is precisely in those contexts that a sense of socially imposed powerlessness and fatalism, among other things, seriously limits individuals' ability to enact personal intentions. In other words, these American HIV-prevention theorists seemed to overlook that "who you are," defined by a particular sociocultural context, explains and determines to a great extent what an individual can and cannot do.

The second point of agreement in the workshop was that, if personal intention is strong enough, behavior follows: "There was general consensus that the intention to perform a given behavior is one of the immediate determinants of that behavior. The stronger one's intention to perform a given behavior, the greater the likelihood that the person will, in fact, perform that behavior" (Fishbein et al., 1991, 5).

While this statement may have some validity for certain individuals or groups, or be a desirable goal of interventions, the reality is that in many individuals risky behavior does coexist with relatively strong intentions to act safely and promote personal health. It is my belief that intentions lead to behavior only where individuals have power and control over the consequences of their behavior, or have enough resources to deal with the negative outcomes or consequences of enacting their intentions. Unfortunately, this is not the case for those groups where HIV is spreading at faster rates in this country: gay men of color, minority women, the young. The positive correlations between intention and behavior noted in the introductory section were found among groups of highly acculturated, mostly-English-speaking

Latino gay/bisexual men; these same studies revealed a strong negative relationship between sexual risk behavior and socioeconomic markers of income and education within the samples (Diaz, 1995).

By placing the causes of HIV transmission in individual behavior, the theorists biased the focus of prevention towards individual responsibility (so true to the American tradition!), minimizing the role of structural and sociocultural determinants. Not surprisingly, theories proposed to date have, with very few exceptions, overlooked the processes—personal, interpersonal, and situational—involved in enactment of intentions in a context of multiple competing factors—including low perceptions of personal control, and fatalism regarding the inevitability of infection, so present in impoverished, powerless, vulnerable groups. As a consequence, the majority of theories have focused on cognitive/perceptual factors—for example, giving more weight to individuals' perceptions of control (such as perceived self-efficacy) than to "real world" determinants or limitations of individual control—over individual health-promoting decisions and behavior. Finally, these models have given little attention to individual or group differences in expression of human sexuality, or to cultural determinants of sexual behavior.

There is obviously need for a "shift of paradigm" in HIV prevention research. We need to develop models that are domain-specific (sexuality and drug use) and that focus on the difficulties that persons, dyads, and communities face in enacting personal intentions. More important, we need models that focus on the breakdown of intentionality, and that are sensitive to the historical, cultural, situational, and contextual variables where (so-called) risk behavior occurs. Of special importance would be an attempt to understand risk behavior not in terms of "deficits" in individuals' knowledge, motivation, or skills, but rather as behavior that may have meaning and be quite rational within a given sociocultural context.

Sociocultural Barriers to the Enactment of Safer Sex Intentions

To understand the factors that compete with the practice of safer sex, I interviewed sixty-two Latino gay/bisexual men in San Francisco during the period November 1992 through June 1993; fifty-three men were interviewed in the context of ten focus groups, and nine in individual in-depth interviews. The men were recruited through establishments, organizations, agencies, and friendship networks, ensuring inclusion of both Spanish-speaking, non-acculturated men and English-speaking, acculturated men. Focus groups and interviews were conducted in either Spanish or English, as appropriate. Approximately half of the sample was Mexican or of Mexican descent; the remainder included eight different nationalities from the Caribbean and Central and South America. One focus group was made up of five *"vestidas"* ("the ones who dress-up", feminine ending *-as*), the collective name for transvestite/transgender persons in the non-acculturated Latino gay/bisexual community. Another focus group included five men who had worked for some time with other gay/bisexual men as health educators and outreach workers in Latino-identified AIDS education/prevention programs in the city.

Focus-group and interview questions were formulated to elicit the following subjective experiences of Latino gay/bisexual men: their developmental and social histories as self-identified gay/bisexual men in Latino communities; their past and current sexual behavior; their perceptions of risk for AIDS infection; their level of commitment to practice safer sex; their perceived difficulties and barriers to safe sex practices; and their major sources of social support, including relations with families and friends, with the Latino community, and with the mainstream gay community in San Francisco.

As expected, men in San Francisco showed a high degree of knowledge about HIV/AIDS, accurate perceptions of risk, and a strong desire to protect themselves and their loved ones and to remain healthy. However, in the presence of substantial knowledge, accurate risk perceptions, and positive intentions, the men reported multiple incidents of risky behavior in risky situations, including multiple partners, prostitution, sex in public environments, use of intoxicants during sexual activity, and instances of unprotected anal intercourse. The most striking element of the focus-group and in-depth interview data, however, was the parallel between, on the one hand, men's experiences growing up as self-identified but closeted homosexuals in the context of their Latino families, and, on the other, the expressed difficulties in the practice of safer sex. There were striking "congruencies" and meaningful relations between the answers given to the two seemingly unrelated questions, "What is it like to be a Latino gay/bisexual man?" and "What is the most difficult aspect of practicing safe sex?"

For example, in response to the first question, men spoke of painful doubts about their masculinity during childhood—doubts raised by a social context in which homosexuality is defined as a "gender" problem (i.e., homosexual men are defined as women in men's bodies, or as not being "real" men) rather than a sexual orientation; the men spoke of the need to prove their masculinity to feel accepted by other boys and participate in an often cruel peer culture. In parallel fashion, in response to the second question, men talked about fears of losing their erections when using condoms and of appearing less than manly, or like a *"loca"* (the cultural equivalent of "queen"). Men often described sexual encounters as events where they could show their masculinity, or experience the masculinity of their partners, through dominant, strong, penetrative practices. For many of these men, sexuality has been constructed, through important developmental experiences, as a place to create and restore a sense of masculinity and macho ideal. Thus, extreme focus on penetration and fear of losing erections, identified as major barriers to safer sex, became clearly meaningful within the sociocultural context of machismo for men experiencing same-sex desires within Latino communities.

Similar parallels between internalized sociocultural values and high-risk practices were found for other identified risk factors. For example, there was a clear and meaningful connection between the too common necessity of achieving family acceptance of homosexuality only through silence ("They know but we can't talk about it"), and the men's problems in talking about sexuality or negotiating safer sex. The strong, prevalent perception that homosexuality "hurts my family" was closely related to a sense of sexual shame and a separation of sexuality and social/interpersonal/affective life, as manifested by frequent sexual activity in the context of illicit, hidden encounters with strangers in public cruising environments.

The focus-group data showed that, among most Latino gay/bisexual men interviewed, unsafe practices were not the product of a "deficit" in HIV/AIDS knowledge, motivation, or skills. Rather, important sociocultural factors and values, internalized through socialization practices and currently reinforced by participation in Latino communities and family life, strongly competed with enacting safer sex intentions.

Based on the San Francisco findings, I have outlined a set of barriers or competing factors to the enactment of safer sex intentions. The barriers are listed under six different headings, with the assumption that they express six internalized sociocultural factors. Thus, the barriers are seen not as personal deficits or shortcomings, but rather as logical outcomes or specific manifestations of socialization processes in the sexual lives of Latino gay/bisexual men.

1. Machismo
   A. An extreme and almost exclusive focus on penetrative sexual practices, to the extent that sex without penetration is not considered sex;
   B. perceptions of low sexual control, where a state of high sexual arousal (*"estar caliente"* or "being hot") is used as a socially accepted justification for unprotected sex and surrender of reflective/regulatory control in sexual encounters;
   C. a perception of sexuality as a favored place to prove masculinity, with the possibility of losing penile erection to be avoided at all costs.

2. Homophobia
   A. A strong sense of personal shame about same-sex sexual desire, to such extent that fear of rejection in sexual encounters takes precedence over health concerns;
   B. serious problems in self-identification as a member of a group at risk, with consequent denial of personal vulnerability to HIV;
   C. feelings of anxiety about same-sex sexual encounters, leading to an increased use of alcohol, drugs, and /or other intoxicants in preparation for sexual activity.

3. Family Cohesion (in the context of close personal involvement with homophobic families)
   A. Closeted lives with low levels of identification with, or social support from, a peer gay community;
   B. minimal influence of normative changes in the gay community on sexual behavior, because families are seen as the main social referent group;
   C. a forced separation between sexuality and social/affective life or relationships, promoting anonymous, hidden encounters in public cruising places.

4. Sexual Silence

A. Problems in talking openly about sexuality, resulting in difficulties with sexual communication or safer-sex negotiation in sexual encounters;

B. increase sexual discomfort with all matters pertinent to sexuality;

C. psychological dissociation of sexual thoughts and feelings, decreasing the likelihood of accurate self-observation within the sexual domain.

5. Poverty

A. Decreased sense of personal control over one's life, leading to fatalistic notions regarding health and personal well-being;

B. increased unemployment, drug abuse, and violence, undermining the consideration of HIV infection as a major, central, or priority concern;

C. situations of financial dependence—such as, living with families, exploitative relations with older men, or prostitution—where personal power for self-determination and self-regulation is seriously undermined.

6. Racism

A. Increased personal shame about being Latino, with serious negative consequences for self-esteem and personal identity;

B. lack of participation in the mainstream gay community and its activities (racist and classist values about personal looks, financial power, and educational achievement, highly prevalent in the mostly white and middle-class gay community, conspire against feelings of belonging and social recognition for gay men of color);

C. racist stereotypes of Latino men as "passionate, dark, and exotic," creating pressure from non-Latino white gay men to practice risky sex.

The first assumption of the psycho-cultural model of risk is that there are factors competing with the enactment of safer sex intentions. While it is possible to identify specific competing factors for any given group of individuals or population, such as "Latino gay men," the strength of the actual competition—the degree to which competing variables actually become barriers—will likely vary among individual members. For example, if fear of rejection competes with the intention to use condoms in a sexual encounter, the actual competing effect of the fear vis-à-vis enactment of the intention will vary according to each individual's sense of loneliness and alienation, and consequent need for human contact, touch, and relationship. Thus it is always important to define competing variables in relation to individuals' needs and meanings within a given sociocultural and interpersonal context.

Moreover, as outlined, competing difficulties or "barriers" to the practice of safer sex must be conceptually linked to the specific cultural context that shaped the sexual development of an individual. That is, there is a need to examine and make explicit the cultural lens through which particular difficulties have become meaningful and logical to the individuals who experience them. In this endeavor, it is of paramount importance, for example, to examine the powerful effects, within the given culture, of gender socialization, and to articulate its relation to both heterosexual and homosexual activity. Similarly, it is important to examine what constitutes the culture's domain of accepted awareness (for example, fathers taking adolescent sons to prostitutes to "prove their manhood") and, conversely, what is culturally defined as shameful and secret (for example, sexual penetration of young effeminate boys by men self-defined as heterosexual). Only through such a cultural lens can expressed and observed difficulties in the practice of safer sex be seen not as deficits in an individuals' knowledge, motivation, or skills, but rather as meaningful behavior within a particular sociocultural context. Prevention programs aimed at and focused on "changing behavior," but not taking into account such deeply internalized cultural meanings, are doomed to failure.

Culture and Self-Regulation

The psycho-cultural model of HIV risk is being developed to address and integrate the impact of cultural regulation and self-regulation on the practice of safer sex. It is important, therefore, to visit constructs of both culture and self-regulation as conceptual foundations for the proposed model.

Cultural Theory

As a developmental psychologist who is an enthusiastic, though limited, consumer of anthropological literature, I am always pleasantly surprised at how "psychological" and "developmental" are anthropologists' definitions of culture. For example, when defining culture, medical anthropologist Cecil Helman (1990) visited both classical (Tylor, 1871) and contemporary (Keesing, 1981) attempts at this elusive definition. Helman concludes, "Culture is a set of guidelines (explicit and implicit) which individuals inherit as members of a particular society, and which tells them how to view the world, how to experience it emotionally, and how to behave in it . . . Culture can be seen as an inherited 'lens,' through which individuals perceive and understand the world that they inhabit and learn how to live within it" (Helman, 1990, 2–3). Because psychologists seek to explain human perception, emotion, and behavior, Helman's definition situates culture at the very heart of their domain.

Culture, providing "guidelines" for perceptions, emotions, and behavior, can be understood as the main, socially shared regulator of cognitive/affective activity, and nowhere are cultural guidelines more powerful and explicit than regarding gender and sexuality, the domains of interest for prevention of HIV among Latino gay men. The majority of cultural groups have explicit guidelines about what constitutes appropriate, valued, or forbidden behavior in sexual communication, extramarital sex, and homosexual activity. Because these guidelines are typically specified in relation to the two different genders, they become internalized as part of a strongly reinforced and deeply ingrained gender socialization process.

Helman's definition is also elaborated along a truly developmental dimension: "Growing up within any society is a form of enculturation, whereby the individual slowly acquires the cultural 'lens' of that society" (Helman, 1990, 3). In development, gender-related sexual guidelines—the social gender—become an integral part of what Helman labels "psychological gender," individuals' gender self-definition in terms of self-perception and sexual behavior. Thus, for most socialized human beings, culturally given guidelines for gender-appropriate sexual behavior become the principal "lens" through which individuals perceive, feel, and act upon their own sexuality.

When current conceptualizations of culture and enculturation are taken into account, the label "psycho-cultural" seems redundant; "cultural" would have sufficed. However, I have decided to keep "psycho-cultural," especially as there are psychologists who still conceptualize culture as outside the domain of psychology—that is, as "outside" the individual. Even though there are some excellent proposals in developmental psychology to develop a truly cultural psychology, most inspired by the work of Vygotsky and cognitive approaches to anthropology (see for example Stigler et al., 1990), these proposals, with very few exceptions, have not yet reached those, in the field of HIV prevention research, interested in theories of health psychology and behavior change.

Self-Regulation

The psycho-cultural model of HIV risk proposed and developed in this chapter is a theoretical framework to aid in understanding problems in self-regulation of sexuality. More specifically, the model aims, as previously noted, to understand the hypothesized breakdown of self-regulatory or volitional functioning in the domain of sexuality among Latino gay men. It is of paramount importance, therefore, to define and discuss the construct of *self-regulation*, as understood in psychology today.

Self-regulation may be formally defined as the human capacity to plan, guide, and monitor one's own behavior "flexibly," in the face of difficult and challenging circumstances (see Diaz et al., 1990; Diaz and Berk, 1992). In self-regulation, the sources of behavioral control are found not in the immediate and external environmental stimuli, but in an internal and self-generated cognitive plan or behavioral intention formulated by the individual to achieve desired goals. Thus, when an individual functions in a self-regulated manner, his or her behavior is guided or regulated not by contingencies (punishments or rewards) in the immediate environment, but by a self-generated plan or behavioral intention possibly quite independent of immediate consequences (expected, imagined, or actual). It is important that many health-promoting behaviors involve immediate personal sacrifice for the sake of long-term positive outcomes and that, therefore, health-promoting behaviors more often than not demand and assume a high self-regulatory capacity and level of functioning.

For developmental psychologists, self-regulation refers to a person's decreasing dependence on external, social, and caregiving structures, and increasing reliance on self-formulated goals and plans, in regulating his/her behavior. Self-regulation is considered a developmental pathway, a movement from other-regulation, signaling a child's increasingly autonomous functioning from caregivers' dictates and external structures. Thus, in developmental psychology, self-regulation is considered not a set of learned skills, but rather a "property" or "quality" of human activity—a level of "functional organization" achieved in development.

Bandura, from a somewhat different perspective, has eloquently written about this quality of human behavior as the capacity for "self-direction":

If actions were determined solely by external rewards and punishments, people would behave like weathervanes, constantly shifting direction to conform to whatever momentary influence happened to impinge upon them. They would act corruptly with unprincipled people and honorably with right-principled ones, and liberally with libertarian and dogmatically with authoritarians. In actuality, except when subjected to coercive pressure, people display considerable self-direction in the face of many competing influences. (Bandura, 1986, 335)

In Bandura's social cognitive perspective, self-regulation involves enactment of three interrelated but distinct and sequentially ordered subprocesses (also labeled "subfunctions"): self-observation, judgmental process, and self-reaction. In his own words, "Self-regulation is not achieved by a feat of willpower. It operates through a set of subfunctions that must be developed and mobilized for self-directed change" (Bandura, 1986, 336). Self-observation refers to individuals' abilities to observe and understand the causes and determinants of their own behavior, including personal, contextual, and situational factors influencing their psychological functioning and sense of well-being. Once personal behavior has been observed, individuals must be able to evaluate it in light of a set of internal standards; the processes involved in this evaluative judgment are labeled the "judgmental subfunction." Finally, individuals must be able, "in self-reaction," to actively respond to their judgmental processes—mostly by creating conditions that motivate desired, and decrease undesired, behavior. According to Bandura, by creating personal incentives—contingent rewards or self-motivators that reinforce valued behavior—individuals manipulate their own person–situation context to facilitate enactment of difficult intentions.

As Bandura's exception ("when subjected to coercive pressure") suggests, self-regulation is limited and, as a level of functioning, can break down in certain coercive circumstances. It is my belief, however, that external coercion (such as peer pressure) is only one of the possible competing circumstances that may contribute to a breakdown of self-regulation. For example, deep emotions originating, and subjectively experienced, within the person, such as overwhelming longing and desire for flesh-to-flesh contact, or extreme fear of embarrassment or rejection, may strongly compete with the enactment of safer sex intentions, posing difficulties similar to external coercion. In fact, for coercion to be effective, the coerced person must have a real sense of personal vulnerability and helplessness; coercion is thus a person–situation variable rather than simply a property of context or situation.

Acknowledging that individuals' intentions must often be enacted in the face of competing circumstances, German psychologists Julius Kuhl and Jürgen Beckmann (1985) have defined self-regulation in terms of protecting an intention from "competing action tendencies"—those factors that compete with and undermine its enactment. Unlike Bandura, Kuhl and Beckmann define self-regulation as inside the domain of volition—that is, the domain particularly concerned, in contrast to cognition and motivation, with intention–behavior relations. Self-regulation is thus defined as the set of processes that protects and maintains an intention until enactment is completed:

Despite the continuous pressure exerted by competing action tendencies, people often stick to the behavioral intention they are currently committed to until the goal is reached. This phenomenon suggests the existence of processes that prevent competing tendencies from becoming dominant before the current goal is reached . . . The terms volitional control, action control, and self-regulation will be used here interchangeably to denote those processes which protect a current intention from being replaced should one of the competing tendencies increase in strength before the intended action is completed. (Kuhl and Beckmann, 1985, 102)

Kuhl and Beckmann's theory of action control defines self-regulation as precisely those processes by which intentions are enacted; central to the enactment of intentions are individuals' actual attempts at protecting their intentions from competing action tendencies. In line with Bandura's theorizing, Kuhl and Beckmann suggest that self-regulation is characterized by individuals' implementation of strategies that modify internal processes (for example, shifting attention), as well as situational/contextual variables (for example, avoiding persons and circumstances that create social pressure), so as to favor and support enactment of a particular intention, until the goal is achieved.

Because the capacity for self-direction or self-regulation is an outcome of human development, we should expect individual differences in ability to self-regulate and exercise self-direction in the face of competing circumstances. However, as both Bandura's and Kuhl and Beckmann's theories suggest, self-regulated functioning (that is, actual self-regulated or self-directed behavior) cannot be understood simply as a property of the individual. Self-regulatory functioning assumes the individual's capacity to act in spite of immediate environmental contingencies, yet, paradoxically, self-regulatory functioning is made possible or enhanced—or seriously limited—by its context. In other words, actual expression of self-regulation in a given situation can be either supported or severely limited by the number and strength of competing variables in the particular person–situation context.

I propose that there may be a complex and compensatory relationship between the strength of an individual's capacity for self-regulation and the strength of the competing factors: for self-regulated behavior to occur, the individual's self-regulatory strength and effort must be greater than the strength of the competing variables. In other words, the self-regulatory effort demanded in a given situation is a direct function of the strength of the competing variables. It follows that, in the relative absence of competing variables, most individuals will be able to enact intentions with little self-regulatory effort, but in extremely difficult circumstances, only those with strong self-regulatory capacity may be able to maintain, protect, and enact intentions.

Two important questions emerge: How can we define self-regulatory strength/effort? And, more important, how can we promote it? In light of current theories of self-regulation, I propose that self-regulatory strength is constituted by two important psychological functions:

1. The individual's capacity for self-observation and for awareness of competing factors, in the enactment of a given intention; and

2. The individual's repertoire of actively constructed strategies to modify the person–situation context in ways congruent with the intention.

In the context of an HIV prevention program (Hermanos de Luna y Sol) targeting Spanish-speaking, mostly immigrant, Latino gay/bisexual men in San Francisco, I have had the opportunity to facilitate the processes of self-observation and strategy construction for the practice of safer sex. In response to the question, "What is the most difficult thing for you in the practice of safer sex?" men in the program have reflected on barriers and obstacles to their consistent condom use. For example, a major barrier articulated by many participants is that use of condoms makes them lose their erections—an event extremely disturbing to many, as it undermines the erotic experience of masculine energy sought in same-sex encounters. Further questioning of the participants led to self-observation that loss of erection is not a result so much of physical sensations as of a learned association of condoms with illness/death/loss from the AIDS epidemic; condoms bring deep emotions of loss and grief, interfering with sexual arousal.

As the facilitator, I have mirrored the expressed barrier to the group, asking, "Imagine you are a counselor or an older brother, and one of your clients or a younger brother has this problem. What would you suggest?" To deal with this particular barrier (fear of erection loss), the men began to construct self-reactive strategies, suggesting, for example, that they could move attention away from the penis and focus instead on specific parts of their partners' bodies providing strong erotic charge—for example, nipples, back of the neck, muscular legs. In other words, participants concluded they could recover sexual arousal if they focused on other "masculine," erotically charged aspects of their partners (or themselves). Their strategy construction underscored the stated belief that focusing attention on erection loss would only further decrease arousal.

It is precisely the processes of self-observation and strategy construction that have been missing from many HIV prevention programs, which simply encourage condom use as a health guideline. Those programs may promote compliance, but not sexual self-regulation. Kuhl and Beckmann's action-control theory postulates that one of the most important self-regulatory strategies for the enactment of difficult intentions is "attention regulation"—that is, the movement of attention from the competing variable to the variables or factors that support enactment. It is interesting that the men from Hermanos de Luna y Sol were, in the domain of sexual activity, spontaneously constructing a culturally appropriate and highly contextualized strategy of attention regulation. The self-observation and strategy construction I have witnessed in Hermanos de Luna y Sol has shown me it is possible to promote sexual self-regulation as an effective tool for HIV prevention in Latino gay/bisexual men.

It is my belief that accurate self-observation, and effective strategic modification of the person–situation context to protect enactment of an intention, is most likely domain-specific. For example, someone might be keenly self-observant and quite an agent of change in the domain of business transactions or the domain of academic success; however, the self-regulatory abilities involved might not transfer simply to the domain of the person's own sexual behavior. In addition, I believe that self-observation and self-directed modification of the person–situation context are not necessarily skills that can be learned through training, but rather psychological functions that must be developed and co-constructed in social collaboration with other community members, as in the example of Hermanos de Luna y Sol. However, deeper discussion of these badly needed interventions that may promote sexual self-regulation is beyond the scope of the present paper.

Outline for a Psycho-Cultural Model of HIV Risk

In outline form, the psycho-cultural model of HIV risk can be stated through ten propositions.

1. In an individual's development, cultural guidelines about gender-appropriate sexual behavior become internalized as personal beliefs and cognitive scripts for sexual activity.

2. Many of these cultural guidelines/beliefs/scripts (for example, "Men can't control their sexual impulses," "Non-penetrative sex is no sex at all") are at odds with guidelines for safer sex practices.

3. Individual members of cultural groups are, however, able to formulate and enact safer sex intentions in a self-regulatory fashion, even when the intentions are not supported by their inter-

nalized cultural guidelines/scripts or by their immediate socio-cultural context.

4. To the extent that safer sex intentions are in competition with internalized cultural guidelines/scripts, individuals need to exercise a higher level of self-regulatory strength.

5. Self-regulatory capacity—defined as the ability for self-observation and strategy construction—is domain-specific, is limited, and varies across individuals.

6. In the face of strong competition—personal, interpersonal, or contextual—against safer sex intentions, there is a possible breakdown of intentional, volitional, self-regulatory functioning. This breakdown of intentionality in sexual activity cannot be described simply as the replacement of the original intention with another more congruent intention.

7. In the case of self-regulatory breakdown, internalized cultural guidelines/scripts take over the regulation of individual behavior, and quite often this occurs with limited self-awareness and with a deep sense of lack of control over the person's own sexual behavior.

8. Because, at times of volition breakdown, sexual behavior is regulated by internalized cultural norms and cognitive scripts, "risky" behavior is subjectively experienced, within the given sociocultural context, as meaningful behavior, and is not necessarily experienced as "risk-taking."

9. The psycho-cultural model assumes the presence of relatively strong personal intentions for safer sex, as well as each individual's initial attempts to enact them, but also notes that, as a result of frequent enactment failure, there is a likely weakening of perceptions of self-efficacy and self-control, with development of a certain felt helplessness/fatalism that undermines future formulation of intentions.

10. The volition breakdown postulated by the psycho-cultural model does not explain all instances of unsafe practices. Some individuals engage, for quite different reasons, in unprotected sex, with full awareness and intentionality. Some individuals also take "calculated risks" in the practice of safer sex, with full awareness of possible negative consequences. The psycho-cultural model is best used to explain unsafe behavior that happens in the presence

of individuals' intentions and personal commitment to practice safer sex. Typically in these situations, individuals are not able to articulate or explain fully why risky behavior actually occurs, and may be puzzled why they are continuing to practice risky sex with the best and strongest intentions not to.

The label "psycho-cultural" underscores the fact that, in human development, cultural values that give guidance and provide structure to social relations become internalized, giving shape to individuals' construction of their sense of self and of their role in the social, interpersonal world—including, of course, their values and perceptions of sexuality and its meanings. Cultural guidelines and proscriptions on behavior—such as what constitutes appropriate and valued male sexual behavior—become transferred or internalized as personal values, mores, and cognitive scripts, which in turn become the main regulators of individual behavior. In short, in line with current sociocultural (especially Vygotskian) perspectives on human development, the psycho-cultural model assumes that inter-personal (social) guidelines become internalized as intra-personal (psychological) regulators.

A major tenet of this psycho-cultural perspective is that, because culture becomes internalized (becomes psychological, so to speak), it can greatly influence individuals in the relative absence of external guidance, support, or reward systems. The psycho-cultural model attempts to describe internalized cultural factors—that is, the cultural scripts found not only in social discourse between individuals but also in the cognitive schemata, values, and perceptions within an individual. The search for "psycho-cultural" variables in the domain of sexuality, therefore, becomes a search for the ways culture has become internalized and manifest in an individual's sexual attitudes, perceptions, and behavior.

The internalization of cultural values and guidelines is not a mere passive transfer of values from the social culture to the individual; rather, it involves active co-construction of values and meaning by the individual, through social discourse and collaboration with more expert members of the culture. This active co-construction, or internalization, of cultural guidelines lets individuals feel these guidelines are their own—and, in a deep sense, they are, given the individuals' participation in constructing them. When socialization and internalization processes have been effective, cultural guidelines of behavior are subjectively experienced as "one's own," as coming from within, with conviction and commitment. This is particularly obvious in many Latino men's elaborate statements, typically expressed with great conviction and personal commitment, of what they consider "manly" behavior.

Even though individuals' behavioral intentions are more easily and probably enacted when congruent with, and supported by, both sociocultural context and internalized cultural guidelines, it is true that many individuals can exercise a high degree of self-direction and self-determination over and above cultural, contextual, and situational determinants. That is why many Latino men can enact safer sex intentions that seem to contradict internalized cultural norms about masculinity (such as "Men cannot control their sexual impulses" or "Losing your erection during sex is the most embarrassing thing"). However, competing cultural constructions of what, for example, constitutes valued male behavior make enactment of safer sex intentions much more difficult—perhaps close to impossible for those men whose sense of self-regulation and self-determination in the domain of sexuality is not well developed. More important, these cultural scripts will be among the main regulators of behavior in a volition breakdown over the practice of safer sex. Generally, individuals are unlikely to be consciously aware of cultural determinants of their behavior, and in response to questions about what happened in a given instance of unprotected behavior, may simply and genuinely answer "I don't know."

The psycho-cultural model of HIV risk builds on Bandura's and on Kuhl and Beckmann's theories of self-regulation. On the one hand, the psycho-cultural model recognizes from current theories that (1) self-regulated behavior can be best defined as a person–situation variable rather than as solely the property of an individual; (2) self-regulatory capacity is based upon individuals' self-observation and consciousness of determinants of their own behavior; and (3) self-regulation comes of individuals' active manipulation or modification of competing factors in the person–situation context in ways that facilitate enactment of a given intention.

On the other hand, the psycho-cultural model expands and builds on current theories in three specific ways: (1) the model suggests the possibility that weakened intentions are not simply replaced by stronger intentions but rather, in the face of strong competing factors, there may be a breakdown of volitional/intentional behavior; (2) the model further suggests that, in the face of a volition breakdown, behavior is no longer regulated by an individual's consciously formulated intention, but rather by highly automatized, routinized, and internalized cultural guidelines; and (3) the model underscores that there is a compensatory relation between individuals' self-regulatory strength and competing circumstances, with a volition breakdown less likely to occur when individuals' self-regulatory capacities and/or efforts are stronger than the factors acting against enactment of a given intention. In other words, little self-regulatory strength is required to enact an intention where competing factors are minimal; thus, in line with Kuhl and Beckmann, we must define true self-regulation as occurring only in the face of difficult and challenging circumstances.

Conclusion: Three Psycho-Cultural Hypotheses about Latino Gay Men

It is my belief that the practice of safer sex is particularly difficult for Latino gay men, for whom, therefore, successful enactment of safer sex intentions will demand a great deal of self-regulatory effort. However, self-observation in the domain of sexuality—the major ingredient of sexual self-regulation—has been seriously limited for Latino gay men, socialized in a context of strong homophobic attitudes and socially imposed silence about gay sexuality. Furthermore, I believe that the homophobia and sexual silence in Latin culture—families, churches, and communities—have promoted a virtual dissociation of sexuality from the interpersonal, rational, and affective lives of many who experience same-sex desires. Such dissociation is perhaps the major obstacle to sexual self-regulation for Latino gay men, because the psychosocial construction of homosexuality as the domain of the secret, forbidden, and shameful has made self-observation in this domain extremely difficult, loaded with deeply felt and poorly understood emotions.

Within the psycho-cultural framework, I have proposed that six sociocultural factors—machismo, homophobia, family cohesion, sexual silence, poverty, and racism—have shaped the psycho-sexual development of Latino gay men in the U.S. I have attempted to specify, for example, how cultural values and social discourse on gender-specific behavior and family relations, as well as oppressive experiences of poverty and racism—rather than personal intention to practice safer sex—have become the main regulators of sexual activity within this group of men, who are at high risk for HIV infection. These sociocultural factors, now internalized, have become competing variables and major barriers to the practice of safer sex, and are hypothesized to weaken self-regulatory control of sexual activity.

Accordingly, I would like to advance three specific hypotheses about the risk for HIV in Latino gay men, which should be verified with further empirical observations:

First, the practice of safer sex is difficult and challenging for Latino gay men, especially in circumstances that challenge or threaten the cultural scripts internalized in their cultural and sexual socialization. For example, if sexuality has been culturally defined as a crucial place to prove masculinity or restore a hurt sense of manhood, contexts and situations that threaten the loss of an erection, perceived as the essence of virility, will be extremely challenging and difficult. Similarly, if Latinos are accepted and welcomed into the mainstream gay community almost only when acting out a "careless, hot, and passionate" stereotype—with sexual regulation and control seen as un-Latino— the Latino gays will likely be frequently coerced into "risky" sexual activity by members of the mainstream culture.

Second, given the diminished opportunities for Latino gay men to self-observe in the domain of sexuality, they are relatively likely to experience a breakdown of self-regulatory processes in the face of increasing challenge and difficulty. A necessary condition for the exercise of self-regulation and self-determination in the practice of safer sex is an individual's awareness of personal, interpersonal, and situational variables that make such behavior difficult or compete with enactment of safer sex intentions. In Bandura's social-cognitive model, self-observation stands as the first, most basic subfunction of self-regulation. In his words, "[p]eople cannot influence their own actions very well if they are inattentive to relevant aspects of their behavior . . . If they want to exert influence over their actions, they have to know what they are doing" (Bandura, 1986, 336).

For the majority of Latino gay men, however, homosexuality has been culturally accepted—or rather, tolerated—only if not mentioned, not called by its name. In my opinion, the lack of social space to name, speak, share, discuss, and critically reflect on one's homosexual behavior and relations (outside of macho boasting about sexual prowess or conquests) has led to a decreased ability to reflect, observe—and, consequently, to regulate—one's sexual activity. The overwhelming majority of Latino gay men, given this cultural homophobia and sexual silence, may not have had socially supported opportunities to self-observe in the domain of sexuality (in the words of one research participant, "We just don't know ourselves sexually"), and, again, this lack of self-observation may lead to decreased ability to self-regulate sexual behavior.

Finally, my third hypothesis is that, when such volitional/self-regulatory breakdown occurs, culturally scripted information, rather than self-formulated intentions or plans of action, become the main regulators and determinants of sexual behavior. In the case of Latino gay men in the U.S., the previously mentioned six sociocultural variables—machismo, homophobia, family loyalty, sexual silence, poverty, and racism—constitute the basic forces that have shaped these psycho-cultural scripts. Because these six factors explain and give meaning to what appears, from outside, simply "risky behavior," a major claim of the present model is that the high occurrence of unprotected sex among Latino gay men has logic and meaning, from the given sociocultural perspective.

Acknowledgments

Sections of this chapter have been published in my book, *Latino Gay Men and HIV: Culture, Sexuality and Risk Behavior* (New York and London: Routledge, 1997), and are included here with permission of the publisher.

References

Amaro, H. (1995). "Love, Sex, and Power: Considering Women's Realities in HIV Prevention." *American Psychologist*, 50:437–47

Bandura, A. (1986). *Social Foundations of Thought and Action: A Social Cognitive Theory*. Englewood Cliffs, NJ: Prentice-Hall.

———. (1994). "Social Cognitive Theory and Exercise of Control over HIV Infection." In DiClemente, R. J., and Peterson, J. L., (eds.), *Preventing AIDS: Theories and Methods of Behavioral Interventions*, 25–59. New York: Plenum Press

Coates, T., Stall, R. D., Catania, J. A., and Kegeles, S. (1988). "Behavioral Factors in HIV Infection." *AIDS*, 2 (Suppl 1), S239–46.

Diaz, R. M. (1995). "HIV Risk in Latino Gay/Bisexual Men: A Review of Behavioral Research." Paper commissioned by the National Latino/a Lesbian and Gay Organization (LLEGO). Center for AIDS Prevention Studies, University of California, San Francisco.

Diaz, R. M., and Berk, L. E. (1992). *Private Speech: From Social Interaction to Self-Regulation*. Hillsdale, NJ: Lawrence Erlbaum Associates.

Diaz, R. M., Neal, C. J., and Amaya-Williams, M. (1990). "The Social Origins of Self-Regulation." In Moll, L. C. (ed.), *Vygotsky and Education: Instructional Implications and Applications of Sociohistorical Psychology*, 127–54. New York: Cambridge University Press.

Fishbein, M., Bandura, A., Triandis, H. C., Kanfer, F. H., Becker, M., and Middlestadt, S. E. (1991). *Factors Influencing Behavior and Behavior Change: Final Report—Theorists' Workshop*. National Institute of Mental Health. Unpublished manuscript.

Fisher, J. D., Fisher, W. A., Williams, S. S., and Malloy, T. E. (1994). "Empirical Tests of an Information–Motivation–Behavioral Skills Model of AIDS-Preventive Behavior with Gay Men and Heterosexual University Students." *Health Psychology*, 13:238–50

Gagnon, J., and Simon, W. (1973). *Sexual Conduct: The Social Sources of Human Sexuality*. Chicago: Aldine.

Helman, C. (1990). *Culture, Health, and Illness*. Oxford: Butterworth-Heinemann.

Keesing, R. M. (1981). *Cultural Anthropology: A Contemporary Perspective*. New York: Holt, Rinehart and Winston.

Kuhl, J., and Beckmann, J. (eds.). (1985). *Action Control: From Cognition to Behavior*. New York: Springer Verlag.

National Commission on AIDS (1992). *The Challenge of HIV/AIDS in Communities of Color*. Washington, DC.

Parker, R. G. (1991). *Bodies, Pleasures, and Passions: Sexual Culture in Contemporary Brazil*. Boston: Beacon Press.

Stigler, J. W., Shweder, R. A., and Herdt, G., (eds.). (1990). *Cultural Psychology: Essays on Comparative Human Development*. New York: Cambridge University Press.

Tylor, E. B. (1871). *Primitive Culture: Research into the Development of Mythology, Philosophy, Religion, Art, and Customs*. London: John Murray.

Chapter Ten

Gendered Scripts and the Sexual Scene

Promoting Sexual Subjects among Brazilian Teenagers

Vera Paiva

In the first decade of AIDS, Brazilian prevention efforts and campaigns directed at the sexual transmission of HIV were based on the concepts "promiscuity," "fear," "death threat," and "the hazardous Other," within an overall strategy of targeting "risk groups." More recently, safer sex (defined as condom use and fewer partners) has increasingly been promoted through face-to-face activities, and many activists and AIDS educators have begun using small-group interventions. Most of these small-group programs have focused on risk reduction and individual responsibility, through interactive information and, in the relatively rare cases where the necessary resources are available, by modeling sexual communication and negotiation skills.

During our ongoing work with young people in São Paulo, we constantly find that social vulnerability compromises the efficacy of AIDS prevention programs. Participants in our workshops are told that HIV is a highly democratic virus—that its transmission modes do not discriminate by race, age, nationality, gender, or sexual preferences. But when they leave the workshops, they find that HIV transmission is in reality more likely to occur within social and cultural contexts that make some people more vulnerable than others. That is, the youth of my city discover in their everyday lives what epidemiology has been showing on large scale for some time: poor people, minorities, the poorly educated, and the disempowered are more vulnerable (see for example Mann, Tarantola, and Netter, 1992; Lurie, Hintzen, and Lowe, 1995; Parker, 1994, 1996). As Altman puts it, "A number of factors will influence the course of the epidemic, of which the biomedical are not necessarily the most important" (Altman, 1994). These realities motivated us to ask the following questions:

- How should an AIDS prevention program address social and cultural factors that shape and regulate "risky" sex?
- How can AIDS prevention programs go beyond a focus on *behavioral change* and *individual responsibility?*

In this article, I will outline the theoretical framework for the AIDS prevention programs around which we have built our interventions—and will try to contrast it with some more traditional approaches that have guided AIDS education and prevention work. My discussion will center around examples and lessons learned from a research and intervention program developed with teenage students at public elementary night schools in São Paulo.[1]

Outline of a Theoretical Framework

We began the prevention program in 1991, using small-group approaches inspired by the AIDS Risk Reduction Model (Catania et al., 1990) and the Brazilian reproductive health movement, as well as our previous research, which had indicated that gender norms are a key cultural factor placing young men and women at risk of unwanted pregnancy and/or HIV.[2] We were soon confronted by the importance of social and economic contextual factors, which had not been considered adequately by most existing HIV risk-reduction models and behavioral change interventions. Our research findings stressed how the sociocultural context where sex occurs, and the lack of accessible contraception and reproductive health options—condoms cost about U.S.$1 each at the time of our study—limit individuals' intentions to practice safe sex.

Our project builds on the tradition of Latin American liberation pedagogy, most widely known through the work of Paulo Freire. We seek to promote citizenship while encouraging sexual agency. We assume that behavioral change, condom use, and safer sex should be *part of* programs working with disenfranchised communities, but *not the exclusive goal* or focus. Central to our framework are four key concepts: (1) the sexual subject (from the Portuguese term *"sujeito"*); (2) consciousness-raising or "conscientization" (from the Portuguese term, *"conscientização"*); (3) gendered scripts and bodies; and (4) the sexual scene.

The main objective in the prevention program is to promote the *"sujeito sexual"* ("sexual subject"). The sexual subject is the agent who regulates his/her own sexual life, coping with the complexity of factors competing in his/her life that can result in either "riskier sex" or "safer sex." In the Brazilian tradition, *"sujeito"* integrates the idea of agency with the idea of citizenship (defined as full participation and influence in our society—something that cannot be taken for granted in Brazil). The *sujeito* is one who takes action, one who enacts. The sexual subject is thus the individual capable of regulating his/her own sexual life—which, in practice, means:

- developing a negotiated relation with the sexual/gender culture, rather than simply accepting them at face value or as given in nature
- developing a negotiated relation with family and peer group norms
- exploring (or not exploring) sexuality independent of a partner's initiative
- being able to say "no" and to have this right respected
- being able to negotiate sexual practices pleasurable to oneself, as long as they are consensual and acceptable to the partner or partners
- being able to negotiate safer sex
- having access to the material conditions to make reproductive and safer-sex choices

One feasible path to promoting sexual subjects builds upon the Freirean tradition and stimulates the group to deconstruct their own sexual scenarios through "consciousness-raising" and "coding and decoding" (Freire, 1993). As the examples below show, in a consciousness-building process, consciousness should be seen as more than "awareness" in a strict psychological and clinical sense or resulting from self-observation intended to change attitudes and behaviors. Instead, we situate the concept of *self* within the social group, as the word *"conscientização"* is used in the Brazilian liberation education tradition (Freire, 1983). We are thus talking not only about "self-observation," "scene observation," and "promoting self-regulation" (Diaz, this volume), but also about citizenship.

In developing our intervention in São Paulo, the importance of *conscientização* became especially evident after the first wave of safer-sex workshops. The students expressed feelings of powerlessness and fatalism when faced with the actual context in which their recently formulated intentions of using condoms would quite likely not be enacted. Their disproportionate social vulnerability in turn tended to ruin their awareness achieved during the workshops:

I can't have a choice, destiny will choose for me, I see what I can do with it afterwards.

AIDS is just another burden, why bother? To survive in this crazy and difficult world, and have some fun with sex is the only right I have.

One way we have responded to this sense of powerlessness and fatalism has been to help participants to de-codify how the sociocultural context regulates their sexual lives, and to highlight how social forces can frustrate individuals' intentions to practice safer sex and control their own sexual lives. At the same time, collaborative group activities, which can contribute to a sense of responsibility, helped participants to work through the puzzling obstacles in individual sexual scenes, and towards acceptable and feasible safer sex.

For example, research has shown that the symbolic construction of AIDS in Brazil has stressed old prejudices, with a morbid and accusatory attitude towards the "evil" practices, or attributed identities, of those infected with HIV (Paiva, 1992; Daniel and Parker, 1993). These ideas can shape each safer-sex scene, with the condom itself often symbolizing accusation, promiscuity, or the like, and thereby becoming an obstacle to safer sex (Paiva, 1993, 1994, 1995). De-codifying and challenging AIDS stigma, which today is linked to the very idea of safer sex and condom use, is thus a key first step. When learning how to use a condom, intervention participants produced their own (alternative) codes by "making art using the condom" (in Portuguese, *"fazendo arte com camisinha,"* which implies both artistic creation and a certain erotic playfulness): music, poems, sculptures, paintings, drama, posters, culinary art, etc., *using* condoms as a creative device. We then de-codified safer sex and AIDS symbolism by looking, collectively, at participants' productions.

In another activity, students also modeled erotic and reproductive body parts from dough, decoding the gendered sex education they had received at home. Through this group activity, they learned about HIV transmission and about reproduction, and by talking about sex through highly concrete body parts rather than through complicated science classes enacted on blackboards, they deconstructed sexist education and gender culture, and explored the pluralism of pleasures and morals. In discussion about communication with partners, and about other obstacles to enacting their risk-reduction intentions, they also created "sexual scenes" through which they decoded gender relations and sexual scenarios, passive/active relations, and the socioeconomic contexts where sex occurs.

Although focused on the specific content of gender and sexual relations, this process built on the transformative approach outlined by Paulo Freire:

The *coding* of an existential situation is the representation of that situation showing some of its constituent elements of interaction. *Decoding* is the critical analysis of the coded situation. Its decoding requires moving from the abstract to the concrete; this requires moving from the part to the whole and then returning to the parts; this in turn requires that the Subject recognize himself in the object as a situation in which he finds himself, together with other Subjects. If the decoding is well done, this movement of flux and reflux from the abstract to the concrete which occurs in the analysis of the coded situations leads to the supersedence (surpass) of the abstraction by the critical perception of the concrete, which has already ceased to be dense, impenetrable reality. (Freire, 1993)

Freire here considers meaningful words and emerging themes as codes—an idea that emerged through his innovative program with illiterate rural workers of the 1960s. Freire's work, like most in the Latin American tradition of popular education, was forged within social movements struggling against poverty and oppression, and was used to understand liberation through popular class alliances against the authoritarian elite in many Latin American countries supporting military dictatorships in the 1960s and 1970s. Access to education and literacy was a crucial step, but could only be fully achieved through valuing popular language (words and syntax) and relevant themes, to break the silence of the poor—and in turn make education meaningful for illiterate teenage and adult workers.

Literacy programs that used emerging words and themes as codes were a successful way to finally give access to reading and writing—

they were designed to de-codify the social context by, for example, learning the letter "X" not through *"xadres"* ("chess"), but through *"enxada"* ("hoe"). As people became organized, popular drama, music, and other popular arts were used, as in the past, to communicate and value their lives, heritage, and collective history. At least partly as a result of such work, illiteracy has decreased significantly in Brazil since the 1960s, while national mass media have unified language practice. Yet it remains true that few study beyond elementary school, and that word of mouth, more than written material, continues to reinterpret all other sources of information and remains perhaps the most powerful means for the spread of ideas and social change.

From the late 1970s and early 1980s, when redemocratization began to emerge in Latin America, other definitions of oppression were included in nongovernmental and community initiatives, and sex and gender identity politics entered the scene. In this kind of politics, where the reproductive rights and AIDS movements may be situated, a new face was given to liberation pedagogy—with workshops and small groups used within health education programs to talk about desire, intimate experiences, and gendered bodies, to de-construct and re-construct identities, and to fight violence and discrimination. In this space, popular education and mobilization movements met small-group psychological interventions. Workshops (which in Portuguese we call *"oficinas"*) with a psychological approach to empowerment—generally meaning individual empowerment—began to be very attractive to an educated middle class, but did not always make sense to disenfranchised rural migrants (the majority of night school students whom we have worked with in São Paulo).

As we learned through our activities and group evaluations, such workshops should be only the first step in a larger program to mobilize nonorganized communities to cope with their social vulnerability to HIV. We now understand safer-sex workshops to be a space for the production of "codes" to result in a collective "thematic investigation" of the sexual and gender cultures shaping AIDS and reproduction.

Three social issues are relevant to the "codes" we are introducing—words and themes, gendered bodies and scripts, and sexual scripts and scenes. The first (most in tune with the liberation pedagogy of the 1960s and 1970s), is how the sociodemographic variables that define poverty—considered as a mix of income, education, and housing—are associated with vulnerability to HIV infection. The second concerns the way social context shapes gender systems. The third focuses on how different Brazilian subcultures define a complementary passive/active sexual system that is a key aspect in Brazilian sexual and erotic scripts and sexual scenes (this chapter will focus mainly on heterosexual scripts among young people).[3] As we live in the 1990s and work in a large metropolitan area, the codes and themes produced by the communities with whom we have worked express a mosaic of values, options, and preferences that can result in divergent organized subgroups even though allied by the same socioeconomic constraints.

Consequently, we assume that adolescence, like sexuality, rather than being a universal and transcultural phenomenon, is modeled by cultural, economic, and political influences that cannot be overlooked when thinking about AIDS prevention projects (Paiva, 1994, 1995). As Janice Irvine states, the "changes of puberty, such as menstruation, breast development, wet dreams, and hair growth, are given meanings by the culture in which the adolescent lives" (Irving, 1994). Cultural identifications such as "race, gender, and sexual identity must be recognized as social categories, not biological variables" (Irving, 1994). In our program, we stress how these social categories will shape and regulate each individual sexual scene, and how they are competing factors faced by everyone (see also Diaz, 1997, and in this volume).

Inspired by the pedagogic use of "theater of the oppressed," by psychodrama techniques, and by the social-science constructionist approach to sexuality, including the ideas of "sexual scripts" (Gagnon and Simon, 1973) and "erotic scripts" (Parker, 1991), we have used the "sexual scene" as an approach to group investigation of both the sexual context and the choices made by individuals in relation to protected sex.

AIDS consciousness and sexual literacy cannot be achieved without coding and decoding "sexual scenes," the social and cultural contexts in which sex occurs. Sexual scripts are enacted in every scene, and are learned very differently depending on whether one is a girl or a boy. Most of the time, nonconscious "gendered scripts" limit the power and agency of the *"sujeito sexual"* (sexual subject), as will be seen.

In the "sexual scene" exercise, the person who tells his/her story (the "main character") can put "on stage" all the elements that build a dramatic scene:

- where he/she is (place and time where sex occurs)
- with whom (partners and relationships)
- doing what (actions during the encounter)
- scripts of the characters (each partner's point of view)
- speech (conversation)
- gestures (communication without words)
- feelings (going to the depths of the mind and body)
- personification or concretization of norms ("invisible presence" of peers, parents, religion, gender or age expectations, etc.)
- personification or concretization of access to condoms (that is, of salary, cost of condoms, health service providers, parents, pharmacies)
- knowledge or lack of knowledge (lack of information, misinformation, or prejudices) about HIV and reproduction
- power balance (possibly different in different scenes)
- rhythm of the scene—slow or hurried

In sum, he/she explores many competing variables that fight for the attention of the *sujeito sexual* within the sexual scene. Sexual negotiation or individual skills are *not* our focus prior to scene investigation. In the following sections, I use examples from experiences with this framework to illustrate the gendered codes through which our participants experienced their sexuality.

The Gendered Reproductive and Erotic Body as a Code

The theme most strongly emphasized among the students was pregnancy. Activities focusing on reproduction were most likely to throw new light on the meaning of sexual scenes and to emphasize the legitimacy of planning (being responsible for) the sexual act. The risk of undesired pregnancy was perceived as much greater than the risk of AIDS—a perception entirely understandable from the point of view of these students.[4] In one girl's words: "I have to think about pregnancy before AIDS. If I get infected with HIV I will die—that's it. If I have a baby, I have to live for me and the baby, and two of us will survive."

The students especially appreciated exercises creating models of the erotic and/or reproductive body parts with a mixture of salt, flour, and water. Admiring their models (mouths, hands, breasts, genitals, female and male complete figures, buttocks, tongues, etc.), they learned how their knowledge about the body was gendered, as well as how much they did not know. Other than the penis, male reproductive organs were never modeled in any workshop, although we conducted more than a hundred with young people and a dozen with teachers. Models of the vulva were also comparatively rare. So, when we would put all the models in the center of the room, we would include a complete male reproductive body made by the facilitator, and sometimes also a vulva, after discussing why they were absent. Penises and breasts were the most frequent objects produced by the students, as they represented both sensual pleasure and reproduction. According to the students, men are expected to know everything about pleasure, including female paths to pleasure—and in fact the men did have a better knowledge of the female vulva than did most of the women. The discoveries made and questions raised through the modeling exercise were manifold. "It was the first thing I wanted to study closely, in magazines and 'live,'" said one young man. "Pee and menstruation comes out from this hole, I think . . . They come both from here . . . Or do we have another orifice I have never noticed?" asked a young girl.

Yet the women were avid to learn about sex; they were more than ready to learn from the most experienced girls about pleasure, including the erotic knowledge shared by the open lesbians, as well as about reproduction and contraception. Men pretended less interest in learning about issues unfamiliar to them, since they were supposed to already be very knowledgeable. They indicated they were not interested in, and did not value, male-male sex/erotic wisdom, but did find young lesbians "exciting." In looking at and discussing the models, both women and men paid much attention to explanations about how HIV could pass from one person to another. Most women knew less than we had expected about reproduction and contraception, but knew more than did the men. "Yes, I know the most dangerous time to fuck; it is when they are having . . . their period, when they bleed," said one young man, reflecting the views of many, while "Great, I learned a lot," exclaimed a young girl, "You speak a language I can understand, this is not English!"[5]

Talking about their gender constructs (codes)—about what they knew, and things they "may or may not know or do"—we began to discuss (de-codify) gender roles and gendered scripts, the "lady-killer/ assertive/macho" man and the "naive/passive or resisting" woman. Buttocks, for example, were frequently made during the modeling exercise, and generally accepted as both sensual and contraceptive. They were also an emerging symbol of the existence of different kinds of pleasure, in both same-sex and heterosexual relationships. It is interesting that, after the AIDS epidemic, "homosexuality" had become known—a new word associated with an old stigma (the passive male)—but "heterosexual" and "heterosexuality" were words that needed explanation in most groups, and generally not part of the students' vocabulary.

When students named the models of vulva and penis and the related fluids, the gendered sexual scripts became rapidly obvious; men gave only "street" names to their models, while women chose what might be described as "family" slang (that is, terms used by parents and children), although they knew and some might use street names as well. The penis had "penetrative" and aggressive names like "stick" ("*pau*"), "baton" ("*cacete*"), or "pistol" ("*pistola*")—and the slang for "sperm" ("*porra*") could be used as a noun synonymous with a "hit" or a "blow" ("*porrada*"). The names of animals were frequently used—"bird," "snake," or "chick" for the penis, "spider" or "butterfly" for the vulva. Female genitals were also called by words representing seduction ("pierced," "pursued," "chased"). There was no name for female vaginal fluids; the young men thought that women had the same "*porra*" they did, but without sperm. Most girls were confused about their vaginal fluids, with "vaginal discharge" ("*corrimento vaginal*") used as a generic name.[6]

When we talked about the reproductive and erotic body, we ended up discussing gender not as a cultural lens oppressive for women only, but also in regard to men's oppression by gender norms and how gendered scripts made it difficult, for both men and women, to think about risks. In the imaginary sexual scenes constructed, acting as if a partner were "dangerous" contradicted the need to be a "stud" or "lady-killer," or a "marriageable" or "desirable" woman, and was even more inconsistent with the idea of "surrendering" to love or passion or with the "impulsive, assertive male." In the end, the students concluded the following were oppressive: for men to need to drink to find courage to take initiative or overcome shyness; for women to want men assertive and aggressive in order to feel valued; for women to not be able to "choose" to say "yes" or "no," or to have to settle for "any man"; for women to have to pretend ignorance, even when men might actually prefer them more assertive in sexual intercourse.

Gendered Scripts and Sexual Scenes

According to gender norms in the subculture of these young people, it is the responsibility of girls faced with possibilities of sex to actively choose the right person and the right moment, to try to "make love with people they love." Female responsibility is thus placed long *before* the sexual encounter. The only skill a young women needs is of saying "yes" or "no" to "this" or "that" partner. The consequences of a bad choice are "natural" and expected. It is a woman's fate to be held responsible for the choice and its consequences, but not her role to be careful about practices. Boys, on the other hand, cannot easily "decide" and "choose" before the act of sexual consummation. To think or select is for the future. The first task is to "relieve" sexual pressure, to be assertive and conquer sexual partners—being a lady-killer is not a simple matter. Men's choice comes after pregnancy occurs—accepting or not accepting responsibility for paternity. For example, in one exercise we asked boys to think about a scene in which their last sexual partner (real—or desired if they had not yet had sex) told them "I am pregnant." In the female groups, we asked the girls to do the same, and the conversations they imagined were always similar to this:

Girl: I need to tell you something. I am pregnant.

Boy: Are you sure?

Girl: I did the test.

Boy: But how do you know the baby is mine?

Girl: You were my only man.

Boy: How can I know for sure if I am the father?

The strongest male reaction possible to this event, since condoms were not used and the baby was not planned, is "The baby is not mine!" In exercise after exercise, somebody would indeed say this, and male participants would stick to it as a symbol of what they felt.

In the girls' group, a girl playing the boy's role in the same scene would repeat the same widely expected phrases. Only 33 percent of men we interviewed in this project said they needed to love a sexual partner to have sex, but 88 percent of the women said love was required. On the other hand, women did not feel they had to love or marry their sexual partner to have a baby, while most men said they needed to love the woman to become a father of her child—but then would, even if it were another's child.

Among both the young men and the young women, responsibility for the consequences of the sexual act was always represented by pregnancy, not by HIV infection. For participants in the sexual scene, the possibility of babies out of an idealized context was more likely than HIV to foster responsibility or provide the incentive for avoiding being overcome by emotions—passion, lust, fear of abandonment or labeling, haste, and so on—emotions themselves symbolic of individual histories entangled with cultural regulations. In the sexual scenes, these factors competed for the subject's attention, breaking his/her volition and intentions. In one young man's words, they "prevent one from thinking or putting a condom on."

Yet the young people would panic at the idea of not having babies. During group meetings, for example, lesbians or "sterile" women (never male figures) are mentioned as specters of infertility. The primary meaning of a baby was not—as the Brazilian elite usually suppose of the poor—to have more arms to work, or to provide support during old age. It was to make up for lack of citizenship and disenfranchisement: "My child will, first of all, have all that I did not have, and than be what I was not or do what I did not do," in a young man's words. The child represents the possibility of a better future—one that, in accord with much social research in Brazil, is perceived as the effort of an entire family rather than as an individual achievement. The child the parent(s) will love and take care of will define and fulfill the future, give meaning to a hard adult life. And this adult life, for the majority, has already begun; the students speak of a youth that passed too quickly, of a life marked by tragic events that take hope away, or by worthless events.[7] For the young men, the right to decide when to have children, and the idea that they too are entitled to this right, are new concepts. They are used to feeling mere objects of women's decisions in this regard—an accurate perception, in some ways, of the female fertility revolution in Brazil, accomplished in large part through birth control pills (and irresponsible mass sterilization)—saying, for example, "She is guilty, she is a traitor, she makes me have an adult life before I wanted or decided to." When we suggested that condom use could give them the ability to negotiate their reproductive life, the young men said this was, in their opinion, the most convincing argument for condom use they had heard during the entire program.

In another study (Paiva, 1995), we found these feelings and responses understood, but not shared, by more educated or higher-income college students of the same age. This research showed that undergraduate students had a more egalitarian gender culture and different paths to adulthood than had the poorer, younger night school students interviewed in the current study. They started to work and to have a sexual life later than low-income, less educated young people—on average, two years later for both men and women.[8] Having children carried different meaning and value in groups of different status. Less than 4.5 percent of students in either group studied were married, but 25 percent of the elementary school students, versus 2 percent of the college students of the same age, "wish to have children within the next two years." This difference was highly significant, and there was no significant difference between males and females in the same group. College men thought and felt the same way as their poorer peers, when confronted with the pregnancy announcement—"Is it mine?"—even though they controlled their feelings and were less likely to act them out; however, college women in the same role-playing exercise would never anticipate, and were quite surprised by, this unspeakable male sentiment. The night school students were more likely to act on their attitude, ending the relationship to escape responsibility and/or guilt, but if they were in more regular or formal relationships, would sometimes try to behave differently. And when they would change roles and play the women, all of the men recognized the women's right to be enraged by their attitude—although the role-playing changed no male night school students' basic attitude and the college men remained more prompted to self-reflection.

College students generally had greater knowledge about reproduction, contraception, and modes of HIV transmission, with no significant gender differences in levels of knowledge and information. Sexual intercourse with anal penetration (a high-risk practice) began earlier for night school students, and 32 percent did not see it as risky, while only 1 percent of college students said it is not. In the work-shops, we learned that anal sex as a means to avoid pregnancy was confused, among night school students, with a supposed efficacy of anal sex to avoid HIV infection—an idea of course absolutely incorrect. And, as described above, the anus was also seen as both sensuous and contraceptive.

College women and men tended to balance decision-making power over sex,[9] and they were more likely to believe their friends often used condoms. Night school students found it significantly more difficult to negotiate condom use than did university students, and 33 percent of night school students, versus 18 percent of the university undergraduates, *never* wanted to tell the partner to use condoms. Among the night school students, relatively higher home income was strongly associated with condom use, which was never associated with race, religion, or district of residence.

Our research showed, in short, that income and education produce different sexual scenarios, different gendered scripts, and different sexual scenes in the same city and among the same age group. This helps to explain epidemiological data showing how disenfranchised people are disproportionally vulnerable to HIV. Prevention programs must address this vulnerability, which cannot be characterized as simply an individual's deficit in knowledge, motivation, or skills, possible to correct through behavioral interventions based on models of individual behavior change. Paraphrasing Diaz (1997 and in this volume), prevention programs aimed at and focused on "changing behavior" (such as social marketing of condoms, or skills-building training sessions), which fail to take into account deeply internalized cultural meanings and socioeconomic contexts, are doomed to fail.

The Sexual Scene as Code, and the Sexual Subject

Throughout the prevention program, using the "sexual scene" to identify the difference between intentions to practice safer sex and actual enactment helped students understand and challenge social and cultural regulations. Along with the "dough exercise" (as the students called it) described above, which enabled them to decode their gendered sexual culture and to actively raise their AIDS and reproduction literacy, linking the ideas of the sexual subject and citizenship to the "sexual scene" was, we found, the best instrument for decoding the obstacles to individual enactment (and self-regulation), as well as to community organizing.

The "sexual scene" program worked primarily through actual scenes from the students' lives, with every element concretized or personified in the scene through group collaboration. Here is one schematic example of the use of the "sexual scene":

<u>Step 1</u>   <u>Step 2</u>
scene observation + self-observation →

<u>Step 3</u>
group processing and collaboration + group mobilization →

<u>Step 4</u>
sexual subject (*sujeito*) + increasing citizenship

Reinaldo, for example, told his scene and staged it, with the help of the group:

I was going to a party, in my young uncle's car. I saw a girl in a black mini-blouse, standing there. I asked: "Where are you going?" She said she was going to meet a guy, but he didn't come. I invited her to a wedding. I said, "I am a family guy." She came . . . We danced the whole night. We began petting . . . I drank. We went outside. We had to come back at 5 A.M. to catch the ride back. When we came back, I was in the back of the car, a little drunk . . . My uncle [was] in the front . . . I opened her zipper, and we had sex. I am dating Mônica now for six months, now we use condoms because of pregnancy, but at that night I did not think of anything . . ."

Talking about this with Reinaldo, the group investigated meanings, identifying and personifying the conflicting factors in these events. Some key elements the group felt important in the scene follow:

Reinaldo and Mônica did not have a *place* to have sex other than a car. He would have had *money* to buy a *condom* (but *not* for *every time*). Yet, at this *hour* there was no place to go buy a condom, and the most important thing was to *conquer* her. The only other thing in his mind was the effect of the *alcohol*. When Reinaldo switched roles in order to act out *her script* in that scene, Mônica would *not think of HIV*, but *only pregnancy*, and she had her period the day before. She would never *spend her salary buying condoms*, but would rather use the money to buy bus tickets [which cost the same] since she was going to work on foot some days, and being late to her night school classes because of budget shortfalls. She *feels bad and guilty* about having sex in a car, with someone else listening. Reinaldo would not. But she was *in love*, he was *handsome*, and there was *no other place to go*. She was in a *hurry* to finish it, as was he; he liked her, and wanted to *relieve his urge. Later, after this first date, if they had begun to have a steady relationship, the scenes would take on other meaning as well as new obstacles.* They would have to find some *moment* in one of their houses [which both have only one bedroom for all family members to share] when nobody would be there, and *make love quickly*, or do it *in dark streets of the neighborhood, as does everybody else.*

The storyteller and the group would de-codify every element in the scene and discuss how to solve the puzzle. Our goal was not simply to train sexual negotiation skills through role-playing, although when a trained "facilitator" was leading the group, we might use a particular scene as a model, acted out and performed differently numerous times, as skills trainers do. But our focus was broader; we were trying to foster group collaboration with the person who offered the narrative, to help him/her, as well as each member of the group, to become a subject of her/his own intentions.

We used self-observation and scene-observation to help the students understand what was individual responsibility and what was a role of context that might be better transformed by social organizing and mobilization—the difference between self-regulation following self-observation, such as deciding for abstinence, and self-regulation plus social agency, such as demanding condom distribution in the health clinic. At the end of workshops, our final question was always "All right, you have the information. Suppose you have decided to choose when to have your child and to prevent an undesired pregnancy, or to protect yourselves against HIV. Is it fair to say that you have the material conditions and support necessary to practice safe sex?"

In response to this question, in 1994 some elementary students involved in the project tested out available services in reproductive health, and in sexually transmitted infection and AIDS prevention and treatment. Their experience brought out striking examples, which they shared with the group, of the precariousness of the public health system in São Paulo, the richest city in Brazil. Some of their stories:

One 20-year-old girl had reached an excellent level of communication with her mother concerning sex and contraception, as a result of this program. The mother and daughter talked and decided that whenever the daughter was ready for sex, she would seek out the health service for medical orientation on contraception before the "first time." When she and her boyfriend made the decision to have sex, she went to the public health center to consult with the doctor and was told "Why don't you just remain virgin? Men do not like women who have already slept with someone," and the like.[10]

She was interviewed on the way out of this consultation by a group of students, and felt furious and impotent. If she were a middle-class college student, she would have changed doctors. What can one do when one depends on a public health clinic? This is part of her and the other students' actual sexual scene and its social and cultural regulations.

One young man, encouraged by the work we did, sought a public family-planning service. He was not admitted to the weekly meeting because "Only women are admitted at these meetings." While consulting a urologist for guidance on contraception and sexually transmitted infections at a different health service, he was kicked out because he "did not have any problem [disease] and was wasting the doctor's time for no reason at all." There was no one in line, the service facility was empty, and the young man left, suspecting racism.

This young man, an active black activist in his Catholic base community, died of kidney insufficiency a year later, after waiting unsuccessfully for a kidney transplant. Given such occurrences, it is not surprising that young men and women prefer to self-medicate, or to deny health problems, rather than to receive mostly bad service from the public health system, where they feel helpless and denied their citizenship. The young man's case was the only point in our program where racism or race was mentioned as a key social- and cultural-regulation variable; otherwise, race never came up explicitly in the group dynamics, and only 0.5 percent of the men and women in our sample said that ethnic background was relevant in considering a sexual partner or a date. The sample included 45 percent white Brazilians, 47 percent black/brown Brazilians, 6.5 percent Asian Brazilians, and 1.5 percent Native Brazilians, but there were no significant differences in attitudes, knowledge, or practices among students from the different ethnic groups, whereas, as already noted, education and income variations did impact these.

A boy and a girl pretended they were a couple to be accepted in the (public health clinic's) "family planning" group, where the doctor (a woman) said the condom was not a reliable method, and recommended only hormonal methods; she also did not know how to put a condom on. The "couple" asked permission to perform the "condom on a cucumber" demonstration they had learned in the workshop, and it was enthusiastically received by the family planning group. The doctor then said that the clinic would have free condoms. The "couple" came back another day, and the nurse said the condoms were there but had passed their expiration date, and that she would not be responsible, although she would give the condoms to them anyway. This clinic had, for months, no condoms available.

Contraceptives and condoms rarely were available in the students' sexual world. The places where they had sex (dark corners, cars, common areas in large buildings, or at home when other family members were temporarily out) led to hurried sexual activity. They shared small household spaces with many others and could not afford motel rooms. There were few contraceptive options, and abortion, which was and is illegal, was referred to as "hell." What resources could these youth draw on for encouragement and support in the radical changes they needed to accomplish—especially with the HIV/AIDS epidemic rapidly increasing among the poor—to avoid unprotected sex.

For a person to be a subject, to feel capable, there is need for experience not separated from day-to-day experience. Being a sexual subject is neither a skill nor a behavior that can be trained in a workshop. It is *reflected experience that generates the subject* and that builds up cognitive structures and levels of functioning more fluid and dynamic than previous ones. If conditions for experimentation are limited by collective forces—social, cultural, economic—that cannot be confronted or conciliated, the feeling of impotence will always be greater than the feeling of power or perceived self-efficacy.

Some youth we have worked with begin their experimentation not through sexual negotiation or individual skills-training, but through initiatives related first and foremost to citizenship: investigating the public health system and services for young people; investigating different sexual networks and subcultures in their neighborhoods; demanding free condoms in the clinics; demanding value-free counseling about STDs, HIV/AIDS, and contraception; creating a play about abortion and reproductive rights; demanding male acceptance in family planning counseling meetings; suggesting that dancing halls distribute condoms as well as alcohol.

The key question we need to address with this approach is how we can promote safer sex without adding another burden to the already heavy fatalism that the youth carry from other "failures," which the elite attempt to ascribe to a "lack of individual enterprise/effort" or (when racist) to congenital "limitations" of *nordestinos* (Northeasterners, who make up the majority of the poor, immigrant population in southeastern Brazilian cities such as São Paulo). Hence the need to go beyond the notions of "natural sex" or "the power of hormones," or description of a universal adolescence or uniform gender culture. Decoding the sexual scene with all its built-in socioeconomic and cultural elements is a path to consciousness-raising (*conscientização*).

Conclusion

The first safe sex workshops we conducted in this community were positively evaluated by participants, teachers, and parents. We were able to confirm attitude changes showing more flexible values concerning sex and/or traditional gender roles, more confidence in the reliability of condoms, and broadening of risk perception. Nevertheless, such changes are not easy to accomplish, and do not guarantee consistent safer sex, as the students reported in the evaluation followup process, where they provided examples of how social-cultural regulations are hard barriers to overcome.

When we collaborate with young people of lower status in practicing safe sex, if we do not examine the social and economic limits of our own proposals (for example, "Use condoms!" "Be healthy!"), the novelty of AIDS becomes no more than a new risk, a new item in a life already marked by one's dealings with adversity, by numerous tragic events, by the violence of everyday life, by financial instability, by other diseases long eradicated from a richer world, by housing problems, and—in Brazilian terms—by lack of citizenship. Nor is it possible to think our task accomplished simply by informing these students about the new risk of AIDS and about safer sex and making them "individually responsible." Understanding that risk perception, perceived self-efficacy, and commitment to change are entangled in social and cultural regulations, we have been able to recognize over the course of our program that, most of the time, risky sex is not an individual deficit or responsibility.

We broadened the traditional focus on behavioral change, focus groups, and marketing approaches—in which the social and cultural context is typically used (by "experts") to plan products and determine the best language to "sell" these products to target populations (in turn allowing the "experts" to create models of behavior change based on measurable outcomes).

Many AIDS prevention programs have used well-intentioned social research to investigate meanings, attitudes, and prevalence of behaviors, and to formulate innovative language to preach condom use and safer sex—desirable outcomes, of course. The problem is how to substitute these outcomes-to-be-modeled with more politicized popular education approaches, in which social and cultural factors are understood and illuminated *from the community perspective*. If social and cultural factors are not challenged, we will neither foster the sexual subject nor decrease the heavy fatalism and powerlessness of isolated individuals facing an impenetrable reality—and the result will be that communities in developing countries will, like the poor and marginalized communities of developed countries, continue to see AIDS as just another burden among the many they already carry.

After observing how AIDS, sexual meanings, power hierarchies, and gendered scripts have been codified, we must de-codify them and highlight the internal contradictions in each sexual culture. These contradictions are the open doors for agency, for individual, and group cultural innovation (Paiva, 1990). We agree that the individual history and the permanent process of transformation we experience, including changes in personal identity, may bring different tones and rhythms to sexual life as we age; the meaning of sex is different at each stage in life, with each type of bond, and with each partner, and depends upon whether one is a woman or a man, feels part of a sexual community or not, is rich or poor (Gagnon and Simon, 1973). But our focus should not be individual responsibility, but the context in which individuals must act. To help disenfranchised young people feel less "clueless," less fatalist, consciousness-building or consciousness-raising must show how both gendered scripts and the socioeconomic context in which sex occurs take away the agency of the individual and the power of the sexual subject.

We worked on this project to encourage AIDS prevention based upon real life, real experience, the language of daily life, the creativity of art and of popular religiosity. We have used real emotions, felt by real people, in real contexts and scenarios, all voluntarily shared— rather than celebrities playing at marketing and trying to "model" safer sex behaviors, as in the Ministry of Health campaigns shown on Brazilian television. Without *"conscientização,"* safer sex workshops are a resource-intensive program that can be successful only with the middle class, which can find the resources and social support to fulfill the program's intentions.

We should insist instead on interactive AIDS education programs in which the educator is more of an instigator of problems and a source of information than a problem-solver. Yet we must assume that our work does not finish at the end of meetings, sessions, or classes. Any experienced activist (or therapist) knows that change depends upon a long course of trials, rehearsals, and challenges against habitual personal and social environments. And in contexts like Brazil, it is not feasible to offer individual counseling and clinical interventions for millions of people, to produce the revolution that we need to stop this epidemic. Similarly, we cannot wait for some vague "empowerment" prior to beginning work on AIDS prevention; we need to do both.

Real AIDS prevention will depend on a new pedagogy and on activist wisdom, rather than on depoliticized models of behavioral change, universal psychological theories, or vague statements about powerlessness. Psychological theories can give many insights, as can the social sciences. But to collaborate with impoverished communities, we need more than clinical approaches, more than generic speeches about health, sermons about condom use. The urgency of this epidemic calls for the less simplistic approaches of liberation pedagogy, and demands political coherence in the implementation of these approaches. In countries like Brazil, as in other countries and communities around the world, it is life-wasting luxury not to derive political action from educational action. It is more effective and faster, from the life-saving standpoint, to consider activism or advocacy *a built-in part of our approach to AIDS education*, encouraging personal power by agents of political action—and in turn encouraging sexual agency.

As Paulo Freire would say, "Turn the question around; while ed-

ucation is not the lever for social transformation, transformation itself is an educational event. Transformation teaches us, shapes and re-shapes us" (Shor and Freire, 1987).

Acknowledgments

Special thanks to Richard Parker, who was a wonderful mentor and friend during the whole project reported on here—and a perfect part-ner for this final version of the text. Thanks also to Sara Skinner, Norman Hearst, Rafael Diaz, Peter Aggleton, and Charles Klein for suggestions on the translation of the text into English and for com-ments on the original version.

Notes

1. São Paulo has over 200,000 night school students. To study in a night school, students must be over fourteen years old. Ninety percent of these students work in a paid job or at home during the day.

2. A short description of the workshop was published in English in "*AIDS Action*," Issue 25, by ARTHAG, London, 1994. The participants are all the night students, fourteen to twenty-one years old, of four different districts in São Paulo. The program consisted of individual interviews, long workshops (five three-hour sessions), group evaluation sessions, individual counseling, and community organizing initiatives. As part of the project, approximately 3,500 older night school students participated in a shorter version (six hours) of this workshop. We have trained teachers and health services providers in these districts.

3. Our reading of these issues draws heavily on the conception of gender and sexual systems as defined by Gayle Rubin (1984), active/passive relations as defined by Peter Fry (1982) and Richard Parker (1991, 1999), and erotic scripts as defined by Richard Parker (1991).

4. As I have already argued elsewhere (see Paiva, 1993), it is irrational to approach sexuality with separate programs, yet in most countries family planning and reproductive health are separate programs from AIDS pre-vention.

5. "Not English" would be the equivalent of "not Greek".

6. For an extended discussion of the gendered language of the body in Brazil, see Parker (1991).

7. In in-depth interviews the students say things like: "Since I was twelve, I have had an adult memory," or "I had a very hard young life for my age of thirteen." When we asked them, to begin the interview "Tell me about your life," the first idea that occurred to most was that they have

nothing to tell us (since we are privileged people from the university). What is important in their lives are bad things, tragic experiences. For the most part, they chose a tragic event to talk about. Only 10 percent of them described their lives as "beautiful," "calm," or "nice."

8. To study how education (highly correlated with income) shapes gender differences in sexual meanings, we compared primary night school students with college students, taking a subsample of young men and women from seventeen to twenty-one years old.

9. No college woman responded "I never decide what to do in sexual intercourse" and no college man responded "I always decide"—the two extreme alternatives. On the other hand, 30 percent of the night school women responded that they "never" decide and 9 percent of the men said "I always decide."

10. We had trained most of the health professionals at this health service, as at many others in the area. But only nurses or social workers, mostly women, would come to the training. We never had a male doctor come to a training session on adolescents, HIV prevention, and reproductive choices.

References

Altman, D. (1994). *Power and Community: Organizational and Cultural Responses to AIDS*. London: Taylor and Francis.

Catania, J. A. et al. (1990). "AIDS Risk Reduction Model." *Health Education Quarterly*, 17 (1):53–72.

Daniel, H., and Parker, R. G. (1993). *Sexuality, Politics, and AIDS in Brazil*. London: Falmer Press

Diaz, R. M. (1997). *Latino Men and HIV: Culture, Sexuality, and Risk Behavior*. New York and London: Routledge.

———. (2000) "Cultural Regulation, Self-Regulation, and Sexuality: A Psycho-Cultural Model of HIV Risk in Gay Men." In Parker, R. G., Barbosa, R. M., and Aggleton, P. (eds.), *Framing the Sexual Subject: The Politics of Gender, Sexuality, and Power*. Berkeley, Los Angeles, and London: University of California Press.

Freire, P. (1993). *Pedagogy of the Oppressed*. New York: Continuum Press.

———. (1983). *Education for Critical Consciousness*. New York: Continuum Press.

Fry, P. (1982). *Para Inglês Ver: Identitade e Política na Cultura Brasileira*. Rio de Janeiro: Zahar.

Gagnon, J., and Simon, W. (1973). *Sexual Conduct: The Social Sources of Human Sexuality*. Chicago: Aldine.

Irvine, J. (1994). "Cultural Differences and Adolescent Sexualities." In Irvine, J. (ed.), *Sexual Cultures and the Construction of Adolescent Identities*, 3–29. Philadelphia: Temple University Press.

Lurie, P., Hintzen P., and Lowe, R. (1995). "Socioeconomic Obstacles to HIV Prevention and Treatment in Developing Countries: The Role of the International Monetary Fund and the World Bank," *AIDS*, 9:539–46.

Mann J., Tarantola, D., and Netter, T. (eds.). (1992). *AIDS in the World*. Cambridge: Harvard University Press.

Paiva, V. (1990). *Evas, Marias e Liliths: As Voltas do Feminino*. São Paulo: Brasiliense.

———. (1993). "Sexuality, Condom Use, and Gender Norms among Brazilian Teenagers," *Reproductive Health Matters*, 1, no. 2, 98–110.

———. (1994). "Sexualidade e Genero num Trabalho com Adolescentes para a Prevenção do HIV/AIDS." In Parker, R. G., et al. (eds.), *A AIDS no Brasil*, 231–51. Rio de Janeiro: Editora Relume-Dumará/IMS-UERJ/ABIA.

———. (1995). "Sexuality, AIDS, and Gender Norms." In Herdt, G., and ten Brummelhuis, H., (eds.), *Culture and Sexual Risk: Anthropological Perspective on AIDS*, 97–115. New York and London: Gordon and Breach.

Paiva, V. (ed.). (1992). *Em Tempos de AIDS*. São Paulo: Summus.

Parker, R. G. (1991). *Bodies, Pleasures, and Passions: Sexual Culture in Contemporary Brazil*. Boston: Beacon Press.

———. (1994) *A Construção da Solidariedade*. Rio de Janeiro: Editora Relume-Dumará/IMS-UERJ/ABIA.

———. (1996). "Empowerment, Community Mobilization, and Social Change in the Face of HIV/AIDS." *AIDS*, 10(suppl 3):S27–S31.

———. (1999). *Beneath the Equator: Cultures of Desire, Male Homosexuality, and Emerging Gay Communities in Brazil*. New York and London: Routledge.

Rubin, G. (1984). "Thinking Sex: Notes for a Radical Theory of the Politics of Sexuality." In Vance, C. (ed.), *Pleasure and Danger: Exploring Female Sexuality*, 267–319. London: Routledge and Keagan Paul.

Shor, I., and Freire, P. (1987). *A Pedagogy for Liberation: Dialogues on Transforming Education*. Westport, CT: Bergin and Garvey.

Afterword

The Production of Knowledge on Sexuality in the AIDS Era

Some Issues, Opportunities, and Challenges

Carlos F. Cáceres

Now more than ever, research on sexuality constitutes a broad and contested field. The emergence of HIV and AIDS, with the consolidation of agendas linked to promotion of sexual health and reproductive rights, has given this research area increasing prominence among academics and funding agencies. Not only has there been a growing demand within the academic community for scientific work in this arena, but, more important, this demand has triggered a transformation of institutional, disciplinary, and political boundaries surrounding the production of knowledge of the sexual, and has involved an increasingly complex array of social actors. Traditional holders of scientific authority on sexuality, such as psychologists and biomedical specialists, have been joined by epidemiologists and researchers within the sociological and anthropological traditions. Among non-academics, activists for women's rights and women's health, alternative sexualities, environmental justice, abortion rights, and AIDS prevention have interacted with lawyers and professional politicians, health-care providers, religious leaders, artists, and the press in a proliferation of new kinds of knowledge that compete over the definition of socio-sexual reality, and over the power conveyed by such an operation. It is inevitable there should be tensions, and several questions must be asked to understand and disentangle them. This chapter discusses issues of epistemology and methodology in relation to sexuality research, as well as questions of hermeneutics and agency. It draws upon ideas developed in the context of recent research on sexual behavior and sexual identity in Peru.

Science and the Construction of
Knowledge of the Sexual

When thinking critically, in the late twentieth century, about science, it is difficult not to consider it an institutional activity having multiple positionings and accomplishing many sorts of objectives. Some of these objectives are more formal than others, and many are actually of a ritual nature. However, the *sine qua non* formal objective of science is, doubtless, the production of knowledge regarding "reality," knowledge intended to inform strategies of change, either by solving or alleviating problems, or by reconstituting the context in which (social) issues and problems are so defined.

In spite of background ideologies that present scientific knowledge as universal, the understandings generated by scientific inquiry are in fact local. This localism is complex and multidimensional, and possible metaphors for "local" go far beyond the literally geographic. Hence, the configurations of proximity or mutual exclusion adopted internationally by networks of scientific institutions, both within and across disciplines, provide only partial illustration of the contextuality of scientific understanding. We live in a world heading towards globalization, but in which globalization by no means eliminates the history and effects of colonialism but instead contributes to its postmodern forms. In such a context, the practice of science, and the structures which support it, reflect and even partially define postcolonialism. The internal logic of what Kuhn (1962) described as scientific paradigms, and identity formation/affirmation processes in the scientific institutions of postcolonial countries, interact with broader postcolonial relations to define science in peripheral countries as a set of practices largely subservient to the interests of more powerful nations and their institutions. Not surprisingly, the use of local scientific knowledge (and perhaps of any scientific knowledge) by policy makers in peripheral countries is relatively rare.

In the last two or three decades, a vast literature in the industrialized West has attempted to construct a new paradigm of the sexual. From the perspective of the sociology of knowledge, this account has posited, following Foucault (1980), the deployment of power within the field of sexuality. This is not the place for a thorough review of this account, but some main features will be highlighted (see also Weeks, 1985). In this view, "sexuality" first emerged as a concept during the nineteenth century. It was conceived as part of human nature and, in consequence, could define boundaries of normality whereby all excluded terrain was cast as psychopathology. Through the work of Freud and twentieth-century sexology, sexuality was redefined into a hydraulic model, with drives and repression leading to neurosis—seen less as psychopathological than as a discontent of civilization (Freud, 1961 [1929]). Subsequent social-constructionist analysis aimed to liberate sexuality of essentialist "drives" or "instincts"; rather than a part of human nature (and hence localizable in the human body or psyche), sexuality was understood as integral to culture and acquired through socialization. Such a view of sexuality constituted a hegemonic social/cultural structure policing the possibilities of the body.[1]

To see sexuality from a social/cultural perspective, and as predominantly socially constructed, has two contradictory consequences. On the one hand, this characterization weakens tolerance-promoting positions such as those describing sexual deviance as resulting from errors of nature and, therefore, deserving of sympathy. On the other hand, it lays the ground for social movements engaged in cultural activism to challenge hegemonic forms of sexuality.

Throughout the 1980s, both the women's movement and the lesbian/gay movement were central in efforts leading to creation of new discourses on gender and sexuality. This ideological climate defined the boundaries of the current official funding policies of many key donors, and was finally sanctioned in the agendas of sexual health and reproductive rights meetings, such as the United Nations–sponsored gatherings in Cairo in 1994 and Beijing in 1995.

The AIDS pandemic has been a key source of international motivation to give greater attention to sexuality in scientific discourse—although, as Gagnon (1988) has suggested, the pandemic generated an approach to sexuality *from the perspective of AIDS*, when a more desirable outcome might have been the reverse. Much early work was undertaken by practitioners, epidemiologists, public health specialists, and social psychologists; only later did sociologists, anthropologists, and other social scientists become involved, following growing certainty that a more complex approach to sexuality was crucial to successful AIDS prevention.

During the fifteen years of the epidemic, public health research oriented to HIV and AIDS prevention in the industrialized West has examined: the prevalence and incidence of HIV infection; risk factors (and protective factors) for HIV infection, and their prevalence; knowledge, attitudes, and behaviors relevant to the evolution of the epidemic; design and evaluation of biological and individual-level behavioral interventions for prevention. Mathematical models focusing on HIV and AIDS incidence, mortality, costs, and the impact of interventions have followed. Studies of the social and cultural contexts of the epidemic, including sexuality studies, have been scarcer, as have been studies of structural and so-called community-based interventions.

The prominence given each issue has varied throughout the AIDS crisis, responding to changes in technical approaches to the epidemic and in the accompanying political discourses. During the existence of the World Health Organization's Global Programme on AIDS, for example, the primary focus of interest shifted as follows:

1. AIDS—symptoms and clinical evolution of disease
2. AIDS—infection and risk factors
3. AIDS—sexual behavior and biological and behavioral interventions
4. Sexuality and AIDS
5. Sexuality and sexual health
6. AIDS—Sexual cultures, and interventions in cultural contexts

Generally, new foci did not supersede previous ones, but led to the establishment of alternative approaches linked, usually, to involvement of new disciplines or to competing perspectives within the original disciplines. As Giami and Dowsett (1996) point out, at least two main approaches to sexual behavior research continue to be used— one focusing on risk behaviors, and reflecting epidemiological concerns, the other focusing on the structure and the social and behavioral organization of sexual activity, reflecting the confluence of alternative social theories in sexuality research.

In Latin America, a region relatively peripheral to the production of scientific knowledge, and without a top-priority AIDS epidemic, much research on HIV/AIDS has seen its role as complementary to that conducted in the industrialized West, filling local gaps in the application of foreign theories. For instance, studies of the prevalence and incidence of HIV infection, or of the prevalence of well-established risk factors for HIV infection, have been the norm. Surveys of AIDS-related knowledge, attitudes, and practices have also been common—but their uneven quality and frequent irrelevance to local contexts have offered compelling testimony of the consequences of poor planning when resources are limited.

Social and cultural studies and community based interventions, which currently offer the best examples of context-sensitive work, have been basically marginal in much of the scientific response to date. In North America, the region with the most studies on AIDS, this marginality has occurred because prevention research funding remains connected to well-established professional networks inclined to define scientific rigor in terms as yet incompatible with most social and cultural approaches.[2] Structural-level interventions, such as those addressing the socioeconomic structure, or the legal bases of power relations between groups, have begun to be considered, but remain under-developed.

Within Latin America, limited though its production of HIV and AIDS-related research has been over the last decade, an important momentum can be observed in the promotion of social and cultural research on sexuality and sexual health; nevertheless, studies examining the cultural bases of sex and sexuality continue to be rare. This relates in part to sources of funding. However, one challenge is the need to produce social and cultural research meeting accepted standards of theoretical and methodological rigor; these standards are still to be defined in this area, but any definition must pay fair attention to local experience. A second challenge lies in the need to maximize the impact of local research on public policy—highlighting the urgency of generating strategies of diffusion and advocacy that will encourage increased utilization of scientific production at local and regional levels.

Looking for a New Paradigm?

Since sexuality has, in modern science, largely been constructed as the object of inquiry of subdisciplines within biomedicine, sexuality research has reproduced the theoretical and methodological commitments of biomedical research in general. Statistical and quantitative paradigms have therefore constituted the default models of much of this inquiry. The *social* scientific tradition, with its alternative *quali-*

tative methodologies, particularly in anthropology and certain schools of sociology, remains largely foreign to academic work in sexuality—given that until recently sexuality was considered determined primarily by biology.[3] Moreover, adequate interdisciplinary channels have not existed for biologists, psychologists, and physicians (particularly psychiatrists) to collaborate with anthropologists or sociologists in sexuality research, even assuming the latter were interested in participating.

Qualitative and quantitative paradigms—it is of interest to note the difference between these *methodological* paradigms and the *theoretical* paradigms of sexuality described above—have often been represented as polar opposites. However, it is less important to describe and catalogue these differences than to stress issues of more direct epistemological and practical consequence. The point is not one of type of data (numeric or non-numeric), or of dimension of reality (quantity vs. quality), but of ways of understanding "scientific inquiry"—that is, what questions are appropriate, and how they should be asked.

Quantitative methods usually have a statistical referent. That is, they rely on sampling theory to suggest that numerical findings from a sample approximate those theoretically obtainable from the population as a whole. The precision of such approximation is believed dependent on a set of attributes (for example, sample size or type of sampling), whereas its accuracy is seen as dependent on other conditions (for example, independence of sampling units). On this basis, questions asked frequently refer, for example, to the proportions of sampling units in certain response categories; the central trends shown by specific variables and by the dispersion of values (for example, means, medians, and variances); or to the degree to which certain response patterns suggest the existence of associations between two or more variables, and possible characteristics of such associations. The questions most often asked in quantitative research are connected to hypotheses derived from specific theoretical paradigms, and are falsified or not by the data. They more often tell us how much, when, and how often events occur than why or how things come to pass.

Qualitative methods, in contrast, are tied more closely to the search for meaning, and have their origins in Western traditions of inductive thought.[4] Their main task is not one of measuring trends or proportions, or of ascertaining the presence or the strength and modality of numeric patterns of association, but of developing a theory about the elements and structure of human discourses and practices connected to constellations of meaning that, in turn, may determine or constitute broader social phenomena. The qualitative tradition seeks depth rather than quantification; most of its data are interconnected words and ideas rather than quantities. That said, representativeness remains a concern, although in some cases qualitative sampling may intentionally select extreme or deviant cases to register privileged points of view. In contrast to more quantitative approaches, qualitative inquiry responds to questions of *how, in which circumstances,* and *why.*

Recent years have witnessed increasing resistance to uncritical application of quantitative paradigms and methodologies, and towards adoption of more qualitative perspectives. Political work promoting the latter has played a key role in constructing hypercritical depictions of the quantitative approach. Yet it remains crucial to move beyond the trap of false opposition and studies employing a mix of currently available techniques, to develop *genuinely new* paradigms for sociocultural research on sexuality.

When designing studies that seek to combine both approaches, it is perhaps simpler to think of qualitative and quantitative techniques as two potentially complementary approaches to the collection and analysis of data. In this way, we may more easily develop a more integrated research paradigm. Thinking of research questions as approachable through a combination of techniques, each able to make a unique contribution, should enable a transdisciplinary focus in which techniques are freed from their institutional and intellectual histories and united for the sake of new modalities of understanding. The meaning of a survey is reconstructed when interpreted by a qualitative technique, or when used to question results from a qualitative study. Similarly, qualitative research moves beyond its traditional boundaries when seeking to explain survey findings or when identifying issues for later exploration using quantitative techniques. Together, the combination of an array of techniques and the standardization of triangulation procedures offer an opportunity for a new paradigm of social and sexual research in which epistemological differences may be reconciled.

In developing countries, the shift towards mixed or qualitative approaches in sexuality research has created special opportunities and challenges. The tension between limited numbers of social scientists working on sexuality or gender on the one hand and, on the other hand, the preeminence of biomedical institutions in the field of reproductive health has resulted in the continued predominance of biomedical professionals in behavioral research on sexuality. As some of this dominant research adopts more socio-anthropological frameworks, largely as the result of encouragement from funders and donors, training gaps become evident. In the total absence of qualitative and interpretive research paradigms in the official curricula for most biomedical professions, this development brings important opportunities for the possibility of (ideally horizontal) interdisciplinary work. It also poses serious challenges, however—not least the difficulty of integrating qualitative approaches into technical and political discussions in which interpretive paradigms are seen as "foreign" and suspicious. Additional problems arise from the well-intended but occasionally cavalier adoption of a theoretical framework not completely understood by the researcher, and less clearly patterned in structure and application than its quantitative counterpart. How these tensions are resolved will depend on a political history of science in these countries that is still to be written.

Some Relevant Issues

What follows is a more detailed consideration of some issues that have arisen during recent social and cultural research on sexuality. The focus is on work with which I have been particularly closely associated in Peru, although it is hoped that many points will have broader relevance.

Sexual Identity

In the context of research on HIV and AIDS, sexual identity offers a typical example of how an overly simplistic conceptual framework has been assumed to reflect reality and therefore been widely, if often inappropriately, utilized to design seroprevalence studies (Parker, 1995). One of my first studies (Cáceres et al., 1991) set out to determine the seroprevalence of HIV infection, and its risk factors among homosexual and bisexual men in Lima. In the course of the study, it became clear that categories such as "homosexual" or "bisexual" were extraneous to most of the men interviewed.[5] There was a very limited correspondence between reported sexual behavior and self-classification as "homosexual" or "bisexual." Similarly, the fact that many men refused to self-classify in any of the categories provided made us think that other labels might be preferred.

In later research (Cáceres, 1992), a greater number of options was offered to respondents as possible labels for sexual identity. Terms such as "gay," "*travesti*,"[6] "*entendido*,"[7] "man," or even "woman" were included. This increased the proportion of respondents comfortable with at least one proposed option and, most important, revealed that a single label might hold different, perhaps even opposite, meanings for different people. For instance, for some very feminine individuals, the term "gay" might signify a *macho* style interpreted as fake, insofar as femininity is considered spontaneous or natural among homosexuals. For others, the term "gay" might signify *travesti* or something very feminine. Yet others might find the term "gay" more positive than "homosexual," as it could imply the celebration of a chosen identity. Conversely, for other men, "homosexual" would be an aseptic and neutral technical term, while "gay" might connote a scandalous character who did not respect himself and was responsible for the stigma affecting homosexuals (Cáceres, 1996).

Such findings not only shed light on the need to study more carefully in the context of HIV prevention, processes of self-definition and labelling, but also made evident the complex matrix of meanings and values that plays a role in the production of homoerotic desire, organizes the social life of the actors involved, and restricts the symbolic space of the possible. My most recent work has utilized ethnoscientific techniques such as free-listing and pile-sorting. Gay-identified men who have sex with men (group A), non-gay-identified men who have sex with men (group B), and men from a general population group (group C) had to list terms for men who are homosexually active, and to provide definitions for each term used. Important variability was found among the three groups, not only in the terms provided, but also in the meanings and positive/negative values assigned to those terms common to two or three groups. Subsequently, men were asked to sort thirty cards, with such terms written on them, into piles of affinity, and to describe what like terms had in common; many of the terms were unknown to group C but were more familiar to the sub-cultures of men who have sex with men. Some words seen as dep-recatory by group C participants held neutral or even positive values in groups A and B. Differences in response between group A and group B depended on the degree of participation of group B members in mainstream gay cultures, as well as their social roles—for example, men engaged in prostitution might know some terms, but tended to distance themselves from those carrying any possibility of self-identification. Social class was also an important source of variability. Overall, the study found considerable variability in the semantic uni-verses of different groups of men. This has important consequences for self-identification, homosexual activity, and social interaction (Cá-ceres, 1996).

Sexual Practices

A similar point concerning oversimplication must be made with re-gard to studying sexual practices. During the 1980s, research on sex-uality relied heavily upon statistical description of sexual practices, insofar as some had been constructed as risk factors for HIV/AIDS. The frequency of certain practices was also considered key to under-standing the sexual reality of larger groups of people. It is, however, important to examine some limitations on the usefulness of survey information on "sexual practices as risk factors" when obtained through responses to questions on, for instance, whether vaginal, anal, or oral sex is practiced, whether a condom is used, and (for oral and anal sex between men) which sex role was taken (insertive and/or receptive). Not only may biases (particularly those known as "recall bias" and "social desirability bias") affect the responses, but the het-erogeneity of specific sexual acts, the variety of ways persons refer to them, and the variability of their contexts, make it difficult to fully understand sexual behavior and risk-taking on the basis of responses to a few seemingly simple questions.

In a recent review of several studies examining risk factors for the sexual transmission of HIV (Cáceres and van Griensven, 1994), it has become evident that to ask about sexual practices using standard bio-medical terms does not adequately take into account the enormous *variety* of practices placed under each label. Nor does it allow for the possibility that anal sex, oral sex, mutual masturbation, or any other practice can be performed in a variety of ways. Similar problems pertain to the measurement of secondary practices that impact the risk posed by the primary practice. These secondary practices include behaviors involving: corporal fluids (e.g., whether or not semen is deposited in condoms, on the body, or in its cavities); the use of drugs before, during, and after sex; and patterns of partner selection (that is, sources of selection and, especially, criteria for selection). An overly superficial focus on sexual practices as defined by medical and behavioral science categories, rather than as understood and enacted by the individuals concerned, will inevitably lead to naive formulations of behavior change and to associated problems for intervention and program development. Further, to map human practices in terms of endless biomedical categories is likely to reinforce the construction of a medicalized body, its parts symbolically defined not only in relation to normal and abnormal (sexual) practices, but also in regard to AIDS behavioral risks (Treichler, 1988).

Theoretically, to transcend such an approach we must focus, in more original and comprehensive ways, on the complex determination of sexual activity. This could be done in various ways.

First, the meanings of sexual activity (and of related risk-taking) must be more thoroughly considered. If many persons continue in sexual practices considered risky from the viewpoint of HIV prevention, this is partly because such behaviors hold emotional meaning for them. Annick Prieur's (1988) seminal study on continued risk-taking among some gay men in Norway was among the first to show how unprotected sex was considered important for emotional proximity and feelings of belonging, and that giving or receiving semen was a key symbolic element in some gay sexual cultures.

Second, the relational context must be considered, particularly with regard to power, shared (or imposed) meanings, and communication elements in negotiation of sexual practices. For widely varying reasons, many persons are unable—or unwilling—to say "no" to unsafe sex. A personal interest in protection against unplanned pregnancy or against STD/AIDS is only one in a constellation of determinants affecting an individual's sexual behavior.

Third, attempts to approach sexual activity from outside the classificatory logic of biomedicine are extremely important. Mapping the sexual language of different groups, including young people, may be a first step towards providing alternative cognitive maps, maps more culturally and contextually specific.

By addressing these three concerns, we may be able to develop a richer representation of how and why sexual acts occur in particular ways. This in turn may lead to better interventions for STD/AIDS prevention.

Methodologically, some other issues are worthy of attention. First, Simon and Gagnon's (1984) interactionist formulation of sexual scripts may be helpful in operationalizing some of the theoretical issues I have mentioned, and offers a powerful approach to the study of sexual interactions; it starts with a consideration of "cultural scenarios" (competing discourses and practices of the sexual), and moves on to consider "interpersonal scripts" and "intrapsychic scripts" as spaces where cultural mandates can be either fulfilled or resisted in the pursuit of change. Second, social network theory may prove useful not only in understanding how universes of sexual partners are constituted, but also in the modeling of the AIDS epidemic and the formulation of AIDS-prevention policies (Laumann and Gagnon, 1995). Third, issues of social desirability and of the interpretability of self-reports on sexual behavior are central not only for baseline assessment prior to design and implementation of interventions, but also for the interpretation of post-intervention behavioral data. Such issues have been addressed by Bolton (1992), who criticizes the Western humanist traditions for the assumption that research-related activities can be successfully isolated from other activities with sexual content, simply by disciplinary mandate.

Psychosocial Factors Related to AIDS

As already stated, many studies relating to sexuality have been motivated by the AIDS epidemic and/or funded by HIV-prevention budgets. Naturally, AIDS has been a referent in many such investigations. The vast majority of public health studies in this area has, however, addressed AIDS through surveys of "technical" knowledge, beliefs, and social psychological constructs—such as attitudes toward the disease, toward sick individuals, toward condoms and safer sex. These surveys of knowledge, attitudes, and practices (KAP), derived from the North American traditions of health education and health psychology, were hegemonic in social and behavioral research related to AIDS policy and HIV prevention during the 1980s.

In Latin America, and possibly in the South as a whole, KAP surveys have been constructed as "typical" AIDS studies, and hence have become very popular. The limited size of needed budgets, particularly when respondents are easily accessible (students or health workers, for example), has helped this process. The surveys' limited utility, however, derives not only from problems associated with the KAP approach itself, but from uncritical assumptions inherent in many Anglo-Saxon psychosocial constructs and measurement scales. Further problems derive from lack of strategic planning in the use of such studies, a phenomenon that unfortunately characterizes much scientific research carried out in developing countries.

During the late 1980s, with an international discourse on AIDS emerging from a more humanist tradition, parallel to new concern with sexual cultures, it became evident that new efforts were under way to analyze some of the issues from a contextual and interpersonal perspective. This new perspective gave special emphasis to understanding cultural scenarios, interpersonal scripts, and intrapsychic scripts. The popularization of this social and cultural approach in many academic settings has—even though its impact is still limited— enriched our understanding of factors affecting the course of the epidemic (Giami and Dowsett, 1996).

Henceforth, broadly "biomedical" understandings of sex and sexuality can be treated as one of many discourses constructing the social reality of AIDS (Treichler, 1992)—one sharing symbolic space with religious discourses on AIDS, but also with homophobia, discrimination against commercial sex, xenophobia, postmodern meta-discursive production by the media, AIDS activism, and artistic responses to the epidemic. Of course, the broader discourses on the body and its possibilities, on health and on death, offer additional sources of complexity in the personal experience of AIDS and the determination of social vulnerability to AIDS.

Impact of Interventions

Some research on sexuality during the last ten years has been conducted in the context of public health interventions to prevent the transmission of HIV and other STD pathogens, as well as to diminish unplanned pregnancy and other sexual health problems. In this field, the randomized controlled trial (RCT) has traditionally constituted the paradigm of intervention research. In the specific case of behavioral interventions, tensions generated by uncritical application of RCT design have led to its questioning in many academic settings.

First, its focus on the individual rather than on the community has been criticized. Traditionally, health education programs have provided "preventive information" to individuals and sought to elicit attitudinal/behavioral changes in them. However most programs—at least, most that *make a difference*—do more than simply address individuals. They aim to affect personal interactions, leaders' judgments, institutional arrangements, and social movements; they seek to promote community mobilization, solidarity, and support by facilitating transformations in group consciousness and in culture. Quantitative questionnaires applied to individuals may not only miss some of these changes, but may fail to make sense of changes that programs bring about. More recently, the logic of community intervention trials (in which an intervention is implemented in, for instance, one or two communities while one or two others are followed-up as controls) has been promoted as an alternative intervention strategy, forcing a broadening of the traditional logic of field and quasi experiments. Finally, the legitimacy of nonintervention controls has long been questioned on bioethical terms.

Another fundamental problem relates to definitions of impact. Every *evaluation* links to paradigms of meaning and value, as well as to the available instruments of measurement. Many existing indicators are quantitative in nature. As such, they may not be suited to the measurement of more qualitative outcomes, including service users' perspectives and the overall quality of care. Still less may they be able to offer insight into the extent specific interventions can bring change in gender inequalities and gender relations, some of the most sought-after outcomes in current formulations of sexual health and reproductive rights.

Serious problems may also be caused by social-desirability bias in data collection in evaluations. Moderate biases at pre-test may become greater in post-intervention surveys, where subjects may want either to be helpful or to avoid reproach. The use of qualitative techniques of data collection, including participant observation, may enable us to triangulate upon these problems. Guba and Lincoln (1981) have promoted the use of what they call "naturalistic evaluation." For the findings of a specific evaluation to be useful, a detailed description of the program's social context is needed; this must include an account of practical decisions taken during project implementation. It is the role of other researchers to evaluate which specific elements of program implementation were most important, and the extent to which those specific conditions can be reproduced.

Postmodern Concerns

Finally, it is necessary to highlight some dimensions of what some would identify as a postmodern critique of the production of knowledge. In a landmark essay, the post-feminist writer Donna Haraway (1991) distances herself from the politics of radical social constructionism:

But we cannot afford these particular plays on words—the projects of crafting reliable knowledge about the "natural" world cannot be given over to the genre of paranoid or cynical science-fiction. For political people, social constructionism cannot be allowed to decay into the radiant emanations of cynicism. (Haraway, 1991, 184)

Similarly, she dissents from versions of postmodernism that pose history as a story Western culture buffs tell one another, and that define science as a contestable text and a power field, in which the content is the form:

This is a terrifying view of the relationship of body and language, for those of us who would still like to talk about "reality" with more confidence than we allow the Christian right's discussion on the Second Coming and their being raptured out of the final destruction of the world. We would like to think our appeals to real worlds are more than a desperate lurch away from cynicism and an act of faith like any other cult's. (Haraway, 1991, 185)

This is not an issue of a right or wrong model with which to approach reality. The idea of an apolitical, neutral science guided by aseptic ideals of human progress harks increasingly as a nostalgic utopia or, worse, a modern tale. Haraway continues:

[O]bjectivity turns out to be about particular and specific embodiment, and definitely not about the false vision promising transcendence of all limits and responsibility: The moral is simple: only partial perspective promises objective vision . . . [Objectivity] is about limited location and situated knowledge, not about transcendence and splitting of subject and object . . . [It] is not about dis-engagement, but about mutual and usually unequal structuring, about taking risks in a world where "we" are permanently mortal, that is, not in "final" control. (Haraway, 1991, 190)

New times signal the need, therefore, to redefine scientific praxis and rigor. It is possible such an attempt implies a persistent and recurrent effort to constitute fluid and dynamic standards of comparability and reference. Positioning ourselves through careful description of the contexts of what we do, and of who we are as persons, provides a reference framework necessary to a logic in which honesty and humility constitute crucial elements.

If the myth of the detached, neutral, objective scientist (who in sexual research is probably best equated to a First World, caucasian, heterosexual male) is to be destroyed, the notion of positioned knowledges must be accepted. Fundamental questions of hermeneutics (for example, who we are as producers of scientific knowledge, what our stakes are in the process, and how our own position influences our research interests, our approaches, our readings of reality, and our interpretation of findings) become key bioethical questions. Knowledge is related crucially to power and practice. Science—perhaps less than we would like, but nevertheless importantly—defines reality and its problems, and suggests priorities for practice. Both its reality-defining power and the ways alternative institutional powers influence it make science profoundly political.

When knowledge on sexuality and sexual health is considered in these terms, and when we as "progressive intellectuals" or "sexual health researcher-activists" position ourselves as political actors with specific stakes in a contested field, the magnitude of possibilities— but also the scope of the efforts needed to change reality—becomes apparent. One such effort is handling the loss of status that scientific knowledge will inevitably suffer in a dynamics of repositioning that relativizes its authority. In such a logic, randomized controls, stubborn fidelity to a rigid method, and any monodimensional notion of objectivity become passé. In an era of theoretical and political change when the advent of new postmodern identities—notably proliferating identities around the sexual, and even around HIV status—is crucial, the challenge of a new sexual science, conscious of its political positioning, and more concretely focused on the development of better possibilities of life and sexual health for all, must be faced.

Acknowledgment

I would like to thank Bonnie Shepard for her insightful comments on an earlier version of this paper.

Notes

1. This "sociological" view of sexuality is not contradictory with its counterparts in psychology examining the ways sexual socialization constructs a personal sexuality that can be the object of psychotherapy, sexual therapy, or other care. The key difference is that in the "sociological" view, such a personal sexuality is not viewed as having any essential nature and is, therefore, not defining of normality.

2. We should not forget, however, that recent theoretical/political developments in public health and the behavioral sciences have promoted the use of modified versions of qualitative anthropological techniques, as well as of social marketing.

3. The seminal work on sexual cultures by social scientists such as Margaret Mead was not considered by its creators as work on sexuality, but as work on culture. At the most, it was considered scientific research on the effects of culture on biologically determined human nature (Weeks, 1985; Vance 1995).

4. It is now recognized that inductive thought is also present in the reconstruction of theory and in other elements of praxis in the quantitative tradition.

5. To illustrate, however, how much this logic can be entrenched in our mentality, part of our research audience thought information on the relative prevalence of exclusive homosexuality and bisexuality could be obtained through our study. This happened even though the sample was not a random group of men who had sex with men in Lima (a random sample, in any event, impossible to recruit).

6. Transvestite. In fact, the cross-dressed characters of the Italian *commedia dell'arte* constituted *travesti* roles. Transvestites in Lima tend to have an urban, working-class background, assume a transgendered lifestyle, and work mostly in hairdressing and/or street prostitution.

7. A good translation of the nuance of *"entendido"* would be "connoisseur." *"Entendido"* constitutes a gay-culture label for men somewhat peripheral to homoerotic subcultures, or who are "passing" insiders.

References

Bolton, R. (1992). "Mapping *Terra Incognita*: Sex Research for AIDS Prevention—An Urgent Agenda for the Nineties." In Herdt, G., and Lindenbaum, S. (eds), *The Time of AIDS: Social Analysis, Theory, and Method*, 124–58. Newbury Park, CA: Sage.

Cáceres, C. (1996). "Male Bisexuality in Peru and the Prevention of AIDS." In Aggleton, P. (ed.), *Bisexualities and AIDS: International Perspectives*, 136–47. London: Taylor and Francis.

Cáceres, C., Gotuzzo, E., Wignall, S., and Campos, M. (1991). "Sexual Behavior and Frequency of Antibodies to HIV-1 in a Group of Peruvian Male Homosexuals." *Bulletin of PAHO*, 25:306–19.

Cáceres, C., and Rosasco, A. (1992). "Determinants of Safer Behavior among Men Who Have Sex With Men in Lima." *Abstracts Book*, VIII International Conference on AIDS. Amsterdam, July 7–12.

Cáceres, C., and van Griensven, G. (1994). "Homosexual Transmission of HIV-1: Review Article." *AIDS*, 8(8):1041–51.

Foucault, M. (1980). *The History of Sexuality*, Vol. 1, *An Introduction*. New York: Pantheon.

Freud, S. (1961 [1929]). *Civilization and its Discontents*. New York and London: W. W. Norton.

Gagnon, J. (1988). "Sex Research and Sexual Conduct in the Era of AIDS." *Journal of the Acquired Immune Deficiency Syndrome*, 1:593–601.

Gagnon, J., and Parker, R. G. (1995). "Conceiving Sexuality." In Parker, R. G. and Gagnon, J. (eds.), *Conceiving Sexuality: Approaches to Sex Research in a Postmodern World*, 3–16. New York and London: Routledge.

Giami, A., and Dowsett, G. W. (1996). "Social Research on Sexuality: Contextual and Interpersonal Approaches." *AIDS*, 10(suppl A):S191–96.

Guba, E., and Lincoln, Y. (1981). *Effective Evaluation: Improving the Usefulness of Evaluation Results through Responsive and Naturalistic Approaches*. San Francisco: Jossey Bass.

Haraway, D. (1991). *Symians, Cyborgs, and Women: The Reinvention of Nature*. New York and London: Routledge.

Kuhn, T. (1962). *The Structure of Scientific Revolutions*. Chicago: University of Chicago Press.

Laumann, E., and Gagnon, J. (1995). "A Sociological Perspective of Sexual Action." In Parker, R. G., and Gagnon, J., (eds.), *Conceiving Sexuality: Approaches to Sex Research in a Postmodern World*, 183–213. New York and London: Routledge.

Parker, R. G. (1995). "Estado de la investigación en sexualidad: Avances y desafíos." In Shepard, B., Valdés, T., and Hernández, I., (eds.), *I Seminario Taller Sudamericano Investigación Socio-Cultural en Sexualidad:*

Prioridades y desafíos, 13–27. Santiago: Equipo de Apoyo Técnico de UNFPA, Oficina para América Latina y el Caribe, Serie Seminarios y Talleres N° 1.

Prieur, A. (1988). "Meanings of Unsafe Sex among Gay Men in Norway." *Abstracts Book*, First International Congress on AIDS Education and Comunication, Ixtapa, Mexico.

Simon, W., and Gagnon, J. (1984). "Sexual Scripts." *Society*, 22:53–60.

Treichler, P. (1988). "AIDS, Homophobia, and Political Discourse: An Epidemic of Signification." In Crimp, D. (ed.). *AIDS: Cultural Analysis, Cultural Activism*, 31–70. Cambridge: MIT Press.

———. (1992). "AIDS and the Cultural Construction of Reality." In Herdt, G., and Lindenbaum, S., (eds.), *The Time of AIDS: Social Analysis, Theory, and Method*, 65–100. Newbury Park, CA: Sage.

Vance, C. (1995). "Social Construction Theory and Sexuality." In Berger, M., Wallis, B., and Watson, S., (eds.), *Constructing Masculinity*, 37–48. New York and London: Routledge.

Weeks, J. (1985). *Sexuality and Its Discontents: Meanings, Myths, and Modern Sexualities*. London: Routledge and Kegan Paul.

Contributors

Peter Aggleton is Professor in Education and Director of the Thomas Coram Research Unit at the Institute of Education, University of London. He has worked internationally in the fields of sexuality and sexual health for over fifteen years. He is the editor of the journal *Culture, Health, and Sexuality* and the series of books Social Aspects of AIDS, published by Taylor and Francis. Most recently, he edited *Men Who Sell Sex: International Perspectives on Male Prostitution and HIV/AIDS* (Philadelphia: Temple University Press, 1999).

Regina Maria Barbosa was trained as a medical doctor and recently completed a doctorate in public health in the Institute of Social Medicine, State University of Rio de Janeiro. She is currently a Research Scientist in the Population Studies Center, State University of Campinas, as well as Coordinator of Women's Health Research Programs at the Institute of Health in São Paulo. She has published extensively on reproductive health and reproduction rights, and, with Richard Parker, is the editor of a collection of essays, *Sexualidades Brasileiras* (Rio de Janeiro: Relume-Dumará, 1996).

Frederick Blose studied social anthropology at the University of Natal. He participated in studies on perceptions of commercial sex work and on truckers in South Africa.

Carlos F. Cáceres teaches at the School of Public Health, Cayetano Heredia University, and is Director of Research in REDESS Jovenes, Lima, Peru. He has carried out extensive research in Peru on HIV/AIDS, sexuality, and sexual health among young people and among men who have sex with men. His major publications include journal articles ("HIV/AIDS in Latin America and the Caribbean: 1995 Update." *AIDS 1996*, Supplement A), book chapters ("Fletes in Parque Kennedy: Sexual cultures among young men who sell sex to other men in Lima," in *Men Who Sell Sex*, London: Taylor and Francis, 1998) and two books in Spanish, *SIDA en el Peru: Imagenes de Diversidad* (Lima: UPCH and REDESS Jovenes, 1998) and *Salud*

Sexual en una Ciudad Joven: Un Programa Comunitario en Salud Sexual con y para los Jovenes (Lima: UPCH and REDESS Jovenes, 1998).

Rafael M. Diaz is a social worker and a developmental psychologist. In 1995, after thirteen years as Professor of Psychology and Education at the University of New Mexico and Stanford University, he joined the faculty at the Center for AIDS Prevention Studies, University of California at San Francisco. His current research aims at identifying sociocultural barriers to safer sex practices in Latino gay/bisexual men, and at developing culturally relevant risk-reduction interventions in this community. He is principal investigator of the NIH-funded project "A Sociocultural Model of HIV Risk in Latino Gay Men," which involves qualitative, quantitative, and intervention design studies in Los Angeles, Miami, and New York City. He is the author of the recent book *Latino Gay Men and HIV: Culture, Sexuality, and Risk Behavior* (New York and London: Routledge, 1997).

Gary W. Dowsett is an associate professor and deputy director of the Australian Research Centre in Sex, Health, and Society at La Trobe University, Melbourne. A sociologist, he has since 1986 been continuously researching the nature and impact of the HIV epidemic on Australia's gay communities. He has worked as a consultant to WHO's Global Programme on AIDS in Geneva, and as an adviser to the United Nations Development Programme and to the Joint United Nations Programme on AIDS (UNAIDS). His international work includes designing a seven-country study of young people and contexts of risk in relation to HIV/AIDS. He has recently been developing training programs in community-based research and qualitative research design. His most recent book is *Practicing Desire: Homosexual Sex in the Era of AIDS*, published by Stanford University Press in 1996.

Mónica Gogna is a sociologist and a researcher at the Center for the Study of State and Society (CEDES) and the National Council of Scientific and Technical Research (CONICET) in Buenos Aires. She is involved in research and training in the field of social sciences and health. Her major publications include "Women in the Transition to Democracy," in *Women in Social Change in Latin America* (UNRISD–ZED, 1990); "Some Reflections on Training in Reproductive Health and Sexuality: The Case of a Regional Program in Latin America" (with Silvina Ramos) in *Women's Health Issues*, Vol. 7, No. 2, 1997; and "Factores psicosociales y culturales em la prevencion y tratamiento de las enfermidades de transmision sexual," in *Cadernos de Saúde Pública*, Vol. 14, Suplemento 1, 1998.

Purnima Mane is Director of Program Planning in the International Programs Division of the Population Council in Washington, D.C. She has a postgraduate degree in social work and a doctorate in women's studies. She worked for over fifteen years in India at the Tata Institute of Social Sciences, Mumbai, where she was associate professor in the Department of Medical and Psychiatric Social Work. Her area of special interest covers gender relations and their linkage with HIV/AIDS—specifically analysis of factors enhancing vulnerability—and the needed policy and programmatic interventions. She has published extensively on women's issues and gender relations, specifically in the context of HIV/AIDS. Before joining UNAIDS, she worked for the WHO's Global Program on AIDS in the Unit for Social and Behavioral Studies and Support. She is a founding editor of the journal *Culture, Health, and Sexuality.*

Dédé Oetomo is Associate Reader in Linguistics and Anthropology and Head of the Social Issues Laboratory at the School of Social and Political Sciences and Postgraduate Program, Universitas Airlangga, Surabaya, Indonesia. He is founder-member of GAYa NUSANTARA, a gay advocacy organization which, among other things, coordinates the Indonesian Network of Lesbian and Gay Organizations.

Herman Oosthuizen is currently a masters degree candidate in the Department of Social Anthropology, University of Natal. His field of specialization centers on informal economic activities. He has done research in fields as diverse as informal settlements, tourism, craft work, and sexual health.

Vera Paiva is Professor of Social Psychology as well as a coordinator of the Nucleus for AIDS Prevention Studies (NEPAIDS), at the University of São Paulo. She has worked extensively with research and prevention programs on sexuality and gender in the field of HIV/AIDS and reproductive health. Her major publications include *Evas, Marias, e Liliths: As Voltas do Feminino* (São Paulo: Brasiliense, 1990) and, as editor, *Em Tempos de AIDS* (São Paulo: Summus, 1992).

Richard Parker is Professor of Medical Anthropology and Sexuality in the Department of Health Policies and Institutions of the Institute of Social Medicine, State University of Rio de Janeiro, and Associate Professor of Public Health in the Sociomedical Sciences Division of the Joseph L. Mailman School of Public Health at Columbia University, New York City, as well as President of the Brazilian Interdisciplinary AIDS Association (ABIA). His major publications include *Bodies, Pleasures, and Passions: Sexual Culture in Contemporary Brazil* (Boston: Beacon Press, 1991) and *Beneath the Equator: Cultures of Desire, Male Homosexuality, and Emerging Gay Communities in Brazil* (New York and London: Routledge, 1999). He is editor, with John H. Gagnon, of *Conceiving Sexuality: Approaches to Sex Research in a Postmodern World* (New York and London: Routledge, 1995), and with Peter Aggleton, of *Culture, Society, and Sexuality: A Reader* (London: UCL Press, 1999). He is also a founding editor of the journal, *Culture, Health, and Sexuality.*

Rosalind Pollack Petchesky is Professor of Political Science and Women's Studies at Hunter College of the City University of New York, and was the founder and international coordinator of the International Reproductive Rights Research Action Group (IRRRAG), a seven-country collaborative project. Her book, *Abortion and Woman's Choice: The State, Sexuality, and*

Reproductive Freedom (Northeastern University Press, 1990) won the Joan Kelly Prize of the American Historical Association, and her numerous articles on feminist theory and reproductive rights have been published in many languages and countries. She is co-editor, with Karen Judd, of IRRRAG's book *Negotiating Reproductive Rights: Women's Perspectives across Countries and Cultures* (Zed Books/St. Martin's Press/Women, Ink, 1998).

Eleanor Preston-Whyte is a social anthropologist who works in the fields of HIV/AIDS, adolescent sexuality and health, women's participation in the informal sector, and gender studies. Her work has focused on KwaZulu–Natal in South Africa, where she is currently Deputy Vice-Chancellor for Research at the University of Natal and a principal investigator in the Africa Centre for Population Studies and Reproductive Health. Major publications include *South Africa's Informal Economy* (ed., with C. Rogerson, Cape Town: Oxford University Press, 1991) and *Questionable Issues: Illegitimacy in South Africa* (ed., with S. Burman, Cape Town: Oxford University Press, 1992).

Silvina Ramos is a sociologist and a specialist in social research and training in medical sociology and reproductive health. She is currently a senior researcher in the Health, Economy, and Society Department at the Center for the Study of State and Society (CEDES) and Academic Coordinator of the masters program in social sciences and health at FLACSO/CEDES in Buenos Aires. She serves as a consultant for international agencies such as the IDB, PAHO, and UNICEF, for foundations including the Ford Foundation, John D. and Catherine T. MacArthur Foundation, and International Planned Parenthood Foundation, and for regional and international women's health networks. Since 1993, she has been co-coordinator of the Regional Program of Social Research, Training and Technical Assistance in Reproductive Health and Sexuality (Argentina, Chile, Colombia, and Peru). Recent publications include "Some Reflections on Training in Reproductive Health and Sexuality: The Case of a Regional Program in Latin America" (with Mónica Gogna), in *Women's Health Issues*, Vol. 7, No. 2, 1997; "Induced Abortion in Latin America: Strategies for Future Research" (with J. J. Llovet), in *Reproductive Health Matters*, Vol. 6, No. 11, 1998; and "Los retos de la salud reproductiva: derechos humanos y equidad social" (with J. J. Llovet, M. Gogna, and M. Romero), in D. Filmus and A. Isuani (eds.), *La Argentina que viene*, Buenos Aires: Tesis Norma, 1998.

Rachel Roberts specializes in the field of public health, particularly in relation to commercial sex work. She is currently a Doctoral Candidate at South Bank University, investigating teenage perceptions related to food and nutritional health.

Michael L. Tan is Associate Professor of Anthropology at the University of the Philippines and Executive Director of Health Action Information Network (HAIN), an NGO. He has been active in sexual health programs concerned with information and education work, as well as in research. His latest book, *Shattering the Myths* (Anvil Publishing, 1997), is about HIV/ AIDS in the Philippines.

Veriano Terto Jr. is a social psychologist, with a doctorate in collective health. He is currently the coordinator for the projects area at ABIA, the Brazilian Interdisciplinary AIDS Association, and a member of the Board of Directors for the Grupo Pela Vidda in Rio de Janeiro, Brazil. He has been involved in gay rights and HIV/AIDS activism for more than twenty years, and has published extensively on homosexuality and the politics of AIDS. With Richard Parker, he is the editor of *Entre Homens: Homossexualidade e AIDS no Brasil* (Rio de Janeiro: ABIA, 1998), a collection of essays about the response of gay and bisexual men to the AIDS epidemic in Brazil.

Christine Varga is a biomedical anthropologist by training. Her interest in Africa was kindled as a U.S. Peace Corps volunteer in West Africa (Sierra Leone) in the late 1980s. She first arrived in South Africa in 1991 to undertake research for her masters degree project on maternal-child health practices among women in northeastern KwaZulu–Natal. She subsequently returned for doctoral research in 1993 and has since stayed on as a consultant and researcher. She is married to an Indian South African mathematician.

Index